T0190283

Register Now for Online Access to Your Book!

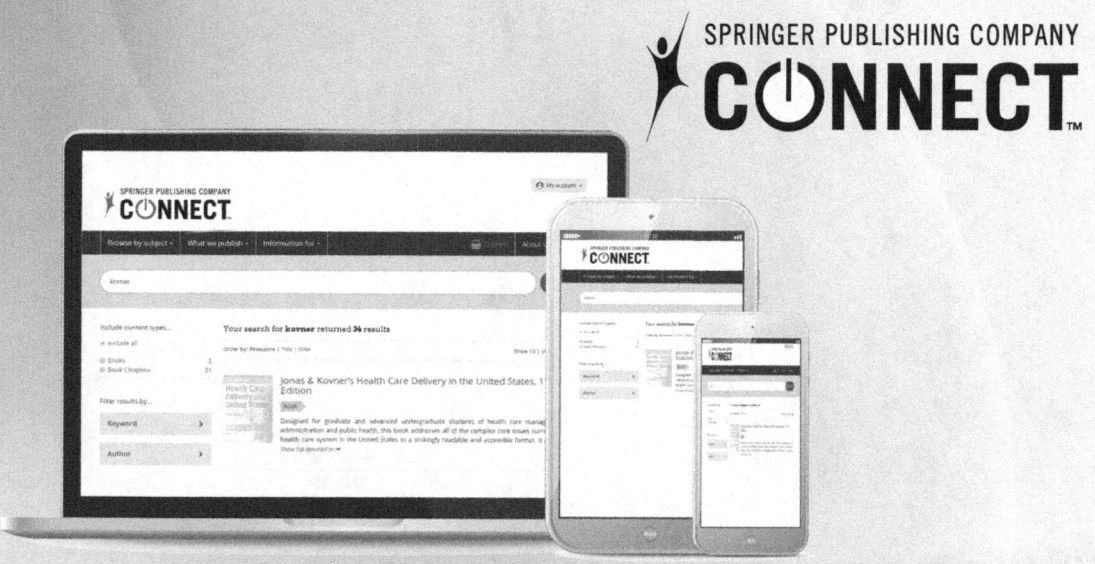

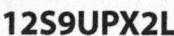

DNP Capstone Projects

Barbara A. Anderson, DrPH, CNM, FACNM, FAAN, is full professor and director of the postmaster's doctor of nursing practice (DNP) program at Frontier Nursing University in Hyden, Kentucky. She has mentored many capstones and dissertations, and is lead editor of *Best Practices in Midwifery: Using the Evidence to Implement Change*, which was awarded an *AJN* Book of the Year (2013). She is coeditor of three editions of *Caring for the Vulnerable: Perspectives in Nursing Theory, Research, and Practice*. The third edition won an *AJN* Book of the Year award in 2012. Dr. Anderson was awarded the 2005 American College of Nurse–Midwives Book of the Year for *Reproductive Health: Women and Men's Shared Responsibility*. Dr. Anderson has served on the editorial board of the *Journal of Midwifery and Women's Health* and currently serves as a journal referee for *Social Science and Medicine*.

Joyce M. Knestrick, PhD, CRNP, FAANP, is associate professor and the online program director at Georgetown University, Washington, DC. She was the associate dean of academic affairs and DNP program director at Frontier Nursing University, Hyden, Kentucky. She has been a nurse practitioner since 1992 and currently practices as a family nurse practitioner at Wheeling Health Right, Wheeling, West Virginia, serving the underinsured vulnerable population in West Virginia. Dr. Knestrick was a pioneer in distance education for nurse practitioners. Her research agenda focuses on the care of low-income and vulnerable populations, particularly in rural Appalachia. She has published and presented locally and nationally on a wide variety of topics related to primary health care, caring for rural and Appalachian populations, and distance nursing education. Dr. Knestrick has received multiple honors and awards, and has served as a reviewer for a number of publishers including Springer Publishing Company, Prentice-Hall, and PRIME. She is treasurer of the American Association of Nurse Practitioners and has been actively involved with the National Organization of Nurse Practitioner Faculties, where she served as the chair of the Distance Education Special Interest Group and coeditor of the *Guidelines for Distance Education and Enhanced Technologies in Nurse Practitioner Education* (2nd edition; 2011). She has chaired multiple DNP capstone projects and served on capstone committees for DNP students from several universities.

Rebeca Barroso, DNP, CNM, is assistant professor at Frontier Nursing University in Hyden, Kentucky. She won the 2011 W. Newton Award from the American College of Nurse–Midwives Foundation to support her replication study on nurse–midwifery burnout. She coauthored a chapter in *Best Practices in Midwifery: Using the Evidence to Implement Change* and served as a copywriter for the book. Dr. Barroso has mentored DNP students at the University of Minnesota and Frontier Nursing University. She is active in the American College of Nurse–Midwives and the Minnesota Advanced Practice Nurses Coalition.

DNP Capstone Projects

Exemplars of Excellence in Practice

Barbara A. Anderson, DrPH, CNM, FACNM, FAAN

Joyce M. Knestrick, PhD, CRNP, FAANP

Rebeca Barroso, DNP, CNM

Editors

SPRINGER PUBLISHING COMPANY

NEW YORK

Springer Publishing Company, LLC
11 West 42nd Street
New York, NY 10036
www.springerpub.com

Acquisitions Editor: Margaret Zuccarini
Composition: S4Carlisle Publishing Services

ISBN: 978-0-8261-3025-9
E-book ISBN: 978-0-8261-3026-6

14 15 16 17/ 5 4 3 2 1

The author and the publisher of this Work have made every effort to use sources believed to be reliable to provide information that is accurate and compatible with the standards generally accepted at the time of publication. Because medical science is continually advancing, our knowledge base continues to expand. Therefore, as new information becomes available, changes in procedures become necessary. We recommend that the reader always consult current research and specific institutional policies before performing any clinical procedure. The author and publisher shall not be liable for any special, consequential, or exemplary damages resulting, in whole or in part, from the readers' use of, or reliance on, the information contained in this book. The publisher has no responsibility for the persistence or accuracy of URLs for external or third-party Internet Web sites referred to in this publication and does not guarantee that any content on such Web sites is, or will remain, accurate or appropriate.

Library of Congress Cataloging-in-Publication Data

DNP capstone projects : exemplars of excellence in practice/Barbara A. Anderson, Joyce M. Knestrick, Rebeca Barroso, editors.
   p. ; cm.
Includes bibliographical references and index.
  ISBN 978-0-8261-3025-9—ISBN 0-8261-3025-9—ISBN 978-0-8261-3026-6 (e-book)
  I. Anderson, Barbara A. (Barbara Alice), 1944– editor. II. Knestrick, Joyce M., editor. III. Barroso, Rebeca, editor.
  [DNLM: 1. Advanced Practice Nursing—United States. 2. Education, Nursing, Graduate—United States. 3. Evidence-Based Nursing—United States. 4. Nurse's Role—United States. 5. Nursing Research—United States. WY 128]
  RT73
  610.73072—dc23

             2014016027

Printed in the United States of America by Gasch Printing.

To the DNP-prepared practitioner who is translating the evidence into practice and creating the future of nursing.

Contents

SECTION I: THE DNP DEGREE AND CLINICAL SCHOLARSHIP

SECTION II: DNP EXEMPLARS: EXCELLENCE IN PRACTICE

Contributors

Barbara A. Anderson, DrPH, CNM, FACNM, FAAN   Professor and Director of Postmaster's DNP Program, Frontier Nursing University, Hyden, Kentucky

Tia P. Andrighetti, DNP, CNM   Associate Professor, Frontier Nursing University, Hyden, Kentucky

Edie Devers Barbero, PhD, RN, PMHNP-BC   Assistant Professor, University of Virginia School of Nursing. Charlottesville, Virginia

Rebeca Barroso, DNP, CNM   Nurse–Midwife, HealthEast Care, Saint Paul, Minnesota, and Assistant Professor, Frontier Nursing University, Hyden, Kentucky

Bobbie Berkowitz, PhD, RN, NEA-BC, FAAN   Dean and Mary O'Neil Mundinger Professor, Columbia University School of Nursing, New York, New York

Linda Cole, DNP, CNM   Nurse–Midwife, Lisa Ross Birth and Women's Center, Knoxville, Tennessee, and Past President, American Association of Birth Centers

Kathleen Flarity, DNP, PhD, CEN, CFRN, FAEN   Emergency Clinical Nurse Specialist/Nurse Scientist, Memorial Hospital, University of Colorado Health, Colorado Springs, Colorado

Lynn Gallagher Ford, PhD, RN, DPFNAP, NE-BC   Clinical Associate Professor, The Ohio State University, Columbus, Ohio

J. Eric Gentry, PhD, LMHC, CAC, CEO   Compassion Unlimited, Inc., Sarasota, Florida

Elizabeth Holcomb, PhD, APRN, FNP-C   Associate Professor, Frontier Nursing University, Hyden, Kentucky

Judy Honig, EdD, DNP   Professor and Associate Dean, Columbia University School of Nursing, New York, New York

Judith A. Kaufmann, DrPH, CRNP   Associate Professor and Director, DNP Program, Robert Morris University School of Nursing, Moon Township, Pennsylvania

Joyce M. Knestrick, PhD, CRNP, FAANP   Associate Professor, Georgetown University School of Nursing and Health Studies, Washington, DC

Pamela Lusk, DNP, RN, PMHNP-BC   Clinical Associate Professor, The Ohio State University College of Nursing, Columbus, Ohio

Bernadette Mazurek Melnyk, PhD, RN, CPNP/PMHNP, FAANP, FNAP, FAAN
Associate Vice President for Health Promotion, University Chief Wellness Officer, Dean and Professor, College of Nursing, Professor of Pediatrics and Psychiatry, College of Medicine, The Ohio State University, Columbus, Ohio

David G. O'Dell, DNP, ARNP, FNP-BC   President, Doctors of Nursing Practice, Inc., Balsam, North Carolina

Kathryn Osborne, PhD, CNM   Professor, Frontier Nursing University, Hyden, Kentucky

Carol Patton, DrPH, RN, FNP-BC, CRNP, CNE   Associate Clinical Professor, College of Nursing and Health Professions, Drexel University, Philadelphia, Pennsylvania

Heather Shlosser, DNP, FNP-BC, PMHNP   Assistant Professor, Frontier Nursing University, Hyden, Kentucky

Gwendolyn Short, DNP, MPH, FNP   Nurse Practitioner, Primary Care Center, University of Minnesota and Associate Professor, Frontier Nursing University, Hyden, Kentucky

Janice Smolowitz, EdD, DNP   Professor and Senior Associate Dean, Columbia University School of Nursing, New York, New York

Gigi Whaley-Pryor, DNP, FNP, APRN   Utah Pain and Rehab, Ogden, Utah

Elizabeth Whitworth, DNP, CNM, FNP   Nurse–Midwife, Carl R. Darnall Army Medical Center, Fort Hood, Texas

Xiao Xu, PhD   Assistant Professor, Department of Obstetrics, Gynecology, and Reproductive Sciences, Yale University, New Haven, Connecticut

Foreword

The American Association of Colleges of Nursing (AACN) was very clear in defining the role of individuals with the doctor of nursing practice (DNP) degree when it endorsed the DNP as the single entry degree for advanced practice nurses in 2004 (AACN, 2004). The association contended that the DNP is a practice-focused doctorate that should prepare clinicians for leadership in evidence-based practice (EBP; AACN, 2006). Despite clarity by the AACN on the preparation and role of the DNP versus the PhD, there remains much confusion and variance in the preparation of individuals in DNP programs as well as the roles that DNP graduates should assume in academia and health care. DNP-prepared clinicians should be the best translators of research evidence into clinical practice and health policy to improve the quality and safety of care as well as reduce health care costs through expertise in EBP change projects, outcomes management, and quality improvement projects. On the other hand, PhD-prepared individuals should be the best generators of rigorous research evidence to guide clinical practice (Melnyk, 2013). However, DNPs and PhDs need to work together with other interprofessional colleagues to rapidly and effectively translate evidence-based interventions supported by research into clinical settings for the ultimate purpose of improving health care quality and patient outcomes.

The United States invests billions of dollars a year in research, yet so little of it is translated to real-world health care settings. Many practices within health care continue to be based on tradition instead of on best EBPs. Although the U.S. Preventive Services Task Force has long published evidence-based prevention recommendations on screening and behavioral counseling that are viewed as "gold standard," these evidence-based guidelines and other evidence-based clinical preventive services by providers are underutilized, which results in wasteful health care spending and, more importantly, loss of life years for Americans (Melnyk, Fineout-Overholt, Gallagher-Ford, & Kaplan, 2012). Research findings that do eventually make it into real-world practice settings often take years or decades. Thus, there is an urgent need for DNP-prepared individuals to speed the translation of research findings into practice to ultimately improve health care and health outcomes. For this to happen more quickly, DNP students must receive an education that prepares them to be the best translators of research evidence into clinical care, education, and health policy. That preparation should include in-depth knowledge and skills building in (a) the EBP paradigm and the steps of EBP; (b) EBP leadership and mentorship of others in evidence-based care; (c) working with clinicians on behavior change to EBP; (d) creating and changing cultures, environments, and systems to support and sustain EBP; (e) how to best influence policy with the best evidence; (f) informatics; and (g) how to successfully conduct EBP change projects, outcomes management, and quality improvement projects that include a rigorous outcomes evaluation.

There are several DNP programs throughout the United States that are requiring students to conduct capstone projects that are original research, which contributes to the ongoing confusion regarding the preparation and role of individuals with the practice doctorate. The capstone project in DNP education should be focused on an EBP change project or quality improvement/outcomes management initiative that aims to enhance health care quality, safety, patient outcomes, or health policy. Stephen R. Covey said "to know but not to do is not to know." When we know the best evidence, it must be quickly implemented in practice and policy. This terrific book fills a needed gap in resources that will greatly assist both faculty and DNP students in planning and conducting appropriate capstone projects. It is filled with outstanding examples of how research-based knowledge can be transferred into real-world settings to improve health care quality and patient outcomes. Various approaches to capstone projects are highlighted with outcomes that were achieved. It is a "must read" for educators and DNP students.

Bernadette Mazurek Melnyk, PhD, RN, CPNP/PMHNP, FAANP, FNAP, FAAN
Associate Vice President for Health Promotion
University Chief Wellness Officer
Dean and Professor, College of Nursing
Professor of Pediatrics and Psychiatry, College of Medicine
The Ohio State University
Columbus, Ohio
Editor, *Worldviews on Evidence-Based Nursing*

REFERENCES

American Association of Colleges of Nursing. (2004). *AACN position statement on the practice doctorate in nursing*. Retrieved November 25, 2012, from www.aacn.nche .edu/dnp/position-statement

American Association of Colleges of Nursing. (2006). *The essentials of doctoral education for advanced nursing practice*. Retrieved November 25, 2012, from http://www .aacn.nche.edu/publications/position/DNPEssentials.pdf

Melnyk, B. M. (2013). Distinguishing the preparation and roles of the PhD and DNP graduate: National implications for academic curricula and healthcare systems. *Journal of Nursing Education, 52*(8), 442–448.

Melnyk, B. M., Fineout-Overholt, E., Gallagher-Ford, L., & Kaplan, L. (2012). The state of evidence-based practice in U.S. nurses: Critical implications for nurse leaders and educators. *Journal of Nursing Administration, 42*(9), 410–417.

Preface

While experiencing unprecedented wealth and high expenditures on health care, Americans are sicker and die sooner than citizens of many high-resource nations. This paradox has been the subject of multiple studies. In comparison to 16 other high-resource nations, the United States ranks highest in adverse birth outcomes, injuries, homicide, adolescent pregnancy, sexually transmitted infections, HIV/AIDS, death from drugs and alcohol, obesity, diabetes, heart disease, chronic lung disease, and disability among the elderly. These findings affect all socioeconomic levels, ethnic backgrounds, and ages (National Research Council and the Institute of Medicine, 2013).

The American health care system is expensive and there are poor health outcomes among our citizens. Further, we are facing a looming crisis of inadequate spaces for preparing nurses in our universities, in spite of high interest in the profession among our people. In response, the nation has imported high numbers of nurses from poorer nations. These nations, having prepared these nurses, now struggle with an inadequate workforce as a result of aggressive recruitment to staff America's health care system (Anderson, 2012). Yet, in the practice arena, our nurses—native-born or immigrant—are restricted in their ability to practice to the full scope of their academic preparation.

Many leaders across the nation, including those in the profession of nursing, are deeply concerned about the underutilization of nursing skills and the barriers to practice. In 2010, the Institute of Medicine released *The Future of Nursing: Leading Change, Advancing Health* (Institute of Medicine [IOM], 2010). This document calls for enabling the nursing profession to practice to the full extent of knowledge and skills consistent with academic preparation (IOM, 2010).

In 2004, the American Association of Colleges of Nursing (AACN) released the position statement advocating for the doctor of nursing practice (DNP) degree, a new terminal degree focusing on the translation of knowledge into clinical practice (AACN, 2004). One way in which this translation of knowledge has been occurring is through the capstone projects of DNP students. The DNP capstone project is a scholarly method to directly impact quality of care and health care outcomes. Translating knowledge into practice and disseminating outcomes for care and policy are consistent with the call for action in the IOM report.

The DNP capstone project has generated much dialogue. Foundational books have been written about the integration of the DNP *Essentials* (AACN, 2006) into the curriculum, the process of developing a capstone project, using evidence-based practice, and disseminating capstone findings. As DNP educators, we have been greatly enriched by this evolving discussion. This book seeks to add to the dialogue by presenting exemplary capstone projects that have provided leadership for change in clinical practice, enhanced interdisciplinary collaboration, promoted advocacy and policy changes, or contributed to quality improvement in health care systems. Each exemplar presented is linked to one or more of the DNP *Essentials*.

It is our hope that this book will, in some small measure, demonstrate the impact of DNP capstones on changing clinical nursing practice, health care, and better outcomes for the people of our nation. To that end, we dedicate this work to the DNP-prepared practitioner who is translating the evidence into practice and creating the future of nursing in our nation.

Barbara A. Anderson
Joyce M. Knestrick
Rebeca Barroso

REFERENCES

American Association of Colleges of Nursing. (2004). *AACN position statement on the practice doctorate in nursing*. Washington, DC: Author. Retrieved from http://www .aacn.nche.edu/dnp/position-statement.pdf

American Association of Colleges of Nursing. (2006). *The essentials of doctoral education for advanced nursing practice*. Washington, DC: Author. Retrieved from http:// www.aacn.nche.edu/publications/position/dnpessentials.pdf

Anderson, B. (2012). The nursing workforce shortage: The vulnerability of the health care system. In M. deChesnay & B. Anderson (Eds.), *Caring for the vulnerable: Perspectives in nursing theory, research, and practice* (3rd ed.). Burlington, MA: Jones & Bartlett.

Institute of Medicine. (2010). *The future of nursing: Leading change, advancing health*. Washington, DC: The National Academies Press. Retrieved from http://www .iom.edu/Reports/2010/The-future-of-nursing-leading-change-advancing-health.aspx

National Research Council and the Institute of Medicine. (2013). *U.S. health in international perspective: Shorter lives, poorer health*. Washington, DC: The National Academies Press.

Acknowledgments

There are many persons and organizations who have contributed to the rapid dissemination of the DNP degree and to the difference this degree is making in the translation of knowledge into clinical practice. We acknowledge the American Association of Colleges of Nursing for the groundbreaking development of this degree and for the clarity of the DNP *Essentials*. We thank the Institute of Medicine for the brilliant and supportive document, *The Future of Nursing: Leading Change, Advancing Health* (2010). We recall the day it was released in October 2010 as the dawning of a new era in nursing leadership. We acknowledge the Doctors of Nursing Practice, Inc., and its president, Dr. David O'Dell, for leadership in promoting the DNP as key to improving clinical practice. Drs. Anderson and Barroso wish to credit Dr. Knestrick for the idea for this book. Special thanks to Dr. Bernadette Melnyk and Dr. Bobbie Berkowitz for support of this project and contributing to this work. We are especially grateful to the best nursing editor any of us have ever worked with, Margaret Zuccarini, who lives and breathes confidence in the ability of nurse writers. Lastly, we want to acknowledge and thank America's nursing educators, who deliver the program and guide DNP students into leadership roles that change health care outcomes for our nation.

SECTION I

The DNP Degree and Clinical Scholarship

We can't solve problems by using the same kind of thinking we used when we created them.

—Albert Einstein

The Emergence and Impact of the DNP Degree on Clinical Practice

Bobbie Berkowitz

EVOLUTION OF PRACTICE

Every profession, at some time in its evolution, confronts its weaknesses, successes, and potential. Rarely do these insights occur simultaneously or evolve in a logical progression: that is, a weakness discovered prompts the development and application of a "better idea." Instead, professions evolve through a combination of individual and collective insight, discovery, competition, collaboration, practice, success, failure, need, and ambition. The evolution of nursing as a practice-based profession guided by critical thinking, scientific evidence, a focus on human response, and social determinants has created a discipline that strives to master multiple domains within the dimension of health. We are clinicians, we are scientists, we are educators, we are policy makers, and we are leaders. As such, our ambition, intellect, and social acuity have driven us toward independence in thought and action. It is no wonder that our clinicians and educators have advocated for and developed the role of expert clinician/practitioner accompanied by a new degree, the doctor of nursing practice (DNP).

A brief examination of professional clinical practice in nursing reveals multiple pathways: clinical practice based on nursing knowledge and medical orders; advanced clinical practice based on expanded diagnostic and treatment knowledge and medical protocol; independently derived clinical diagnosis and treatment for primarily well populations; and independent management of medically complex populations. Nursing, a profession with humble roots, has transformed itself many times into a multipurpose discipline. Our clinicians provide a global society with basic to complex management of health and disease across the lifespan in all settings, including home, community, ambulatory clinics, and highly intensive health care environments. Nurse scientists have generated new knowledge for clinical interventions, prevention strategies for population health, including the transmission of infections acquired in hospitals; tools to support nursing decisions; and quality-improvement strategies drawn from discoveries in the domains of health services, comparative effectiveness, policy, and law.

We might assume that today's graduates of schools of nursing face fewer impediments to continued evolution in nursing. History shows that we have faced significant challenges in gaining independence over our practice, education, and science. However, we must not forget how long it has taken to assume a place where our practice, education, and science are represented and respected at universities and health systems throughout the world, including research-intensive academic health centers, federal research institutions, and scientific academies such as the Institute of Medicine (IOM). At the same time, it should be noted that independence and respect are not enjoyed by all advanced practice registered nurses (nurse practitioners) equally across the United States. We know all too well that variation exists across the country in terms of regulatory oversight of practice. Nevertheless, progress for the development of the DNP role is moving quickly.

DEVELOPMENT OF THE DNP ROLE

Less than a decade ago, the American Association of Colleges of Nursing (AACN) proposed that the education of the advanced practice nurse occur at the doctoral level (AACN, 2004). The genesis of a practice-focused doctorate was in part prompted by a series of reports developed by the IOM: *To Err Is Human: Building a Safer Health System*, 1999; *Crossing the Quality Chasm*, 2001; and *Health Professions Education: A Bridge to Quality*, 2003. These reports drew attention to health care-related errors, fragmentation in the health care system, and the need for all health professionals to deliver patient-centered quality care.

The opportunity for nursing to step forward with solutions to the challenges outlined in these three reports was articulated in the *AACN Position Statement on the Practice Doctorate in Nursing* (2004). The AACN position statement examined how the profession could transform both practice and care delivery to achieve higher clinical quality and address serious population health issues such as chronic disease, health disparities, aging, and the application of evidence-based health promotion and prevention interventions. The report detailed 13 recommendations that set in motion the development of today's practice doctorate emphasizing enhancements to master's preparation for advanced practice.

The AACN position statement also outlined the essential areas of content now known as *The Essentials of Doctoral Education for Advanced Nursing Practice*. The *Essentials* include scientific underpinnings for practice; advanced nursing practice; organization and system leadership/management, quality improvement, and system thinking; analytic methodologies related to the evaluation of practice and the application of evidence for practice; utilization of technology and information for the improvement and transformation of health care; health policy development, implementation, and evaluation; and interdisciplinary collaboration for improving patient and population health care outcomes (AACN, 2004, pp. 14,15).

Within the last decade, the educational focus for the DNP has expanded to include competencies in addition to advanced comprehensive clinical care across the lifespan. These additional competencies include leadership, strategy, advocacy, interdisciplinary collaboration, scholarship for quality improvement, and the translation of evidence into practice. Educators and practitioners alike have spent considerable time assuring medical colleagues and members of the public that DNP education will lead to clinical outcomes for patients, communities, and systems that are a superior "product."

In fact, we have argued that advanced clinical nursing care should be provided by practitioners who practice to the full extent of their education and scope of practice, without regulatory or system impediments. This was a focal point of the IOM report, *The Future of Nursing: Leading Change, Advancing Health* (2010). This key message was based on concerns that unnecessary and burdensome restrictions on practice would only exacerbate the critical shortage of primary care providers. In addition, the IOM Committee examined the literature on quality outcomes from advanced practice nurses and cited numerous examples of equal or superior clinical practice compared to their physician counterparts.

Newhouse and associates (2011) conducted a systematic review of care provided by advanced practice registered nurses (nurse practitioners [NPs]) in the United States to compare teams that included NPs to those without NPs. The review covered a period of published literature between 1990 and 2008. Following established inclusion criteria and a grading of the evidence, the review elicited 107 studies. The review considered care provided in community, inpatient, nursing home, and ambulatory surgery settings. Outcomes were analyzed by practice specialty and included NPs, certified nurse–midwives, and clinical nurse specialists. The overall results indicated that care provided by NPs in collaboration with physicians is ". . . similar to and in some ways better than care provided by physicians alone for the populations and in the settings included" (p. 18). The authors concluded that ". . . Nurse practitioners provide safe, effective, quality care to a number of specific populations in a variety of settings" (p. 19).

VARIATIONS AND CHALLENGES

We now have a cadre of DNP-prepared practitioners in a variety of settings across the United States. Over 217 U.S. universities now have DNP programs, and enrollment has increased from 170 students in 2004 to 11,575 students in 2012 (AACN, 2013). This is good news. However, we have challenges ahead. First, we have multiple variations on the definition of advanced practice. As universities developed DNP programs, role emphasis varied by how the content for each of the seven *Essentials* was interpreted. While a number of schools have developed DNP programs that focus on clinical NP education, many have chosen to develop nonclinical advanced roles in leadership, policy, public health, and education. All DNP programs adhere to *The Essentials of Doctoral Education for Advanced Nursing Practice* (AACN, 2006), but the educational mission around this role varies a great deal.

Is variation of the role problematic? That remains to be seen. As the graduates of DNP programs enter the workforce, their ability to articulate their "advanced practice" role to employers and colleagues and to translate their impact on the outcomes expected from practice will be critical. These experiences will provide insight into the public's acceptance and understanding of what value DNP preparation as a leader, educator, policy and data analyst, or advanced practice clinician brings to the health system, organization, or clinical environment.

Dunbar-Jacob, Nativio, and Khalil (2013), in their review of DNP education, provided clear examples of DNP education for roles focused on health systems, primary care, and academia, as well as how these roles are utilized in Pennsylvania. The majority of the DNP graduates from the eight Pennsylvania programs that provide DNP education were prepared for the administration role. The second-largest group was the NP focus.

Dunbar-Jacob and colleagues (2013) encountered a slow adoption of the bachelor's of science in nursing (BSN) to DNP program, and these authors predict that the greatest impact of the DNP role will be in acute care settings in administrative roles. The authors concluded that in the long run the quality of DNP programs will depend on the availability of qualified faculty and providing added value from the master's graduate. The public is just beginning to understand the NP role even though it has been practiced for decades; will they understand an advanced role for nurses focused on the health system?

It should be noted that the recommendation from the AACN to migrate education for all NPs in the future to the DNP level rather than master's level by 2015 has received significant debate. Commentary on the topic was featured in *Nursing Outlook* in the May/June 2011 issue. Commentators were invited to respond to an article by Cronenwett et al. (2011) that expressed concern about the migration of all NP programs to the DNP level. The authors argued such a move would be detrimental to the public.

We will not know the number of schools of nursing that comply with the AACN recommendation for several more years. Some predict that the majority of schools will migrate to the educational requirement of a DNP for the NP, but this remains to be seen. The concern, of course, is that this ongoing debate within the profession poses additional complexity as we educate the public, health providers, and health system executives that NPs are an important solution to expanding the provision of primary care.

A second challenge relates to our capacity to teach the growing number of individuals who pursue the DNP degree. For example, as preparation of NP transitions from the master's degree to the DNP degree, the intensity of time and talent required for a highly complex curriculum including capstone or portfolio requirements and a pre- or postdoctoral residency will stress the capacity of a limited pool of qualified faculty. Should our DNP nurse practitioner programs require DNP-prepared nurse practitioner faculty? Should our DNP nurse practitioner faculty be required to practice so they remain current in evidence-based practice? The way we think about these questions could lead to new standards for educators of DNP programs and could create a shortage of DNP program faculty.

The third and perhaps most critical challenge is the development of the metrics that will help us measure the contribution DNP-educated nurses make to clinical outcomes. The idea that the public should expect a standard of quality from their health care providers should not be a far reach. Yet the literature shows that there have been serious gaps between what we consider "ideal care" and the actual care individuals receive. This revelation, outlined in *Crossing the Quality Chasm* (Institute of Medicine [IOM], 2003), was shocking in the prevalence of care that was not evidence-based and did not follow standard treatment guidelines.

ACHIEVING CLINICAL VALUE

In response to the growing concern about the quality of health care, one of the major purchasers in the health care system, Centers for Medicare and Medicaid Services (CMS), has launched a number of programs. These programs are designed to assist health care providers, including advanced practice nurses, in understanding quality and measuring quality processes and outcomes.

The Patient Protection and Affordable Care Act of 2010 (United States Department of Health and Human Services, 2010) prompted additional quality initiatives mandating, for example, that quality be a factor in physician fee schedules for Medicare payments by 2015 (Medicare FFS Physician Feedback Program/Value-Based Payment Modifier). This measure could effectively link cost and quality in payment policies in order to prompt quality in the system through incentives to provide value to the public.

This Medicare program collects data on provider performance on a range of clinical measures and provides feedback on performance comparisons across health care systems and providers. One of the outcomes of this program will be a payment system that reimburses providers based on "value" instead of "volume." This Medicare initiative known as "value-based purchasing" is detailed in the report, *Roadmap for Implementing Value Driven Healthcare in the Traditional Medicare Fee-for-Service Program* (Centers for Medicare & Medicaid Services [CMS], 2009). The CMS Roadmap outlines the goals for a value-based purchasing system for health care. The goals include: financial viability, payment incentives, joint accountability across the system, effectiveness of care provided, assuring access to care, safety and transparency, transitions across systems, and the meaningful use of electronic health records (EHRs). The complexity of the requirements of these programs to manage and report data, including systems to collect, assess, and utilize measurement data, can be overwhelming for providers and health care systems.

Medicare is not the only purchaser who has developed payment systems based on quality and value. Private insurance markets are equally concerned that they avoid paying for poor quality. As a result, most insurers are implementing quality initiatives in order to reward efficiency and effectiveness (National Committee for Quality Assurance, n.d.).

An important aspect of value-based payment systems that reward quality and create disincentives for poor performance are measurement sets that can be applied to a broad range of practice and provider types and clinical processes and outcomes. Most of the measures utilized in value-based payment systems are endorsed by the National Quality Forum (NQF) through a consensus process (NQF, 2013). The process assures that each measure meets certain standards before it is utilized for quality reporting. The measures undergo rigorous scientific and evidence-based reviews with input from consumers, health care industry leaders, and providers. As of July 2013, the NFQ is host to more than 600 standardized measures that meet criteria set out in the report, *Measurement Evaluation Criteria* (2013). The criteria for endorsed standards include: the standards are publically available, the measure is regularly updated to account for clinical innovation, the measure is intended for performance improvement and accountability, the measure has been tested for reliability and validity, and each measure has been harmonized with related measures.

What does this all mean to current and future DNP-prepared advanced practice nurses? First, health systems, including provider practices, are consolidating in order to create the necessary infrastructure and develop the capacity to manage the complexity needed to meet the growing expectations from the public, purchasers including private and government-funded organizations, and the intent of the Patient Protection and Affordable Care Act of 2010. Second, the need to engage in the process of continuous innovation around clinical care requires access to large and complex data sets populated with patient data in EHRs and linked to other practices and systems through Health Information Networks (HINs). Third, the future of quality health care will depend on a patient-centered, team-based system that provides comprehensive primary and specialty care across the patient's life.

It is unreasonable to expect the future DNP-prepared practitioner will manage care without ready access and knowledge of the systems and requirements for practice. The future practitioner will be faced with complex health systems, complex payment systems, high demand for quality and innovation, and accountability for practice outcomes. The DNP of the future will need to focus on those imperatives necessary to create an environment that embraces this rather daunting new system of care.

IMPERATIVES FOR THE FUTURE

We must be diligent in precisely defining the roles a DNP graduate is prepared to assume and why. How will the nurse with a DNP emphasis in education provide superior education; why should a hospital system hire the DNP-prepared nurse executive; how will a public health department benefit from the DNP-prepared nurse with specialty in population health; and what enhancements in clinical practice can we expect from the DNP-prepared NP?

We are shifting from master's preparation for these advanced roles to doctoral preparation, and it is not enough to assume clinical care, leadership, education, and public health practice will benefit. We must be able to articulate evidence that supports the premise that the DNP is what we need for advanced practice. In other words, what is the value proposition for a student to spend the time and money on a doctoral degree for roles that have been performed by master's-prepared nurses with evidence of good outcomes?

The capstone project component of the DNP education is, of course, one of the methods we use to understand the evidence and outcomes from DNP education. The capstone is one of the exemplars of the value added and should serve as evidence that the role and outcomes are different from master's preparation for advanced practice. This book contains examples of excellence in various DNP practice roles. Chief among how we might learn from these examples is their fit with the chosen new practice role.

Equally important is the fit of the new practice role with the needs of the populations we serve as nurses. What does society require for quality health care in terms of practice, scholarship, and value, and what will society require in the future? It is hard to argue that a leading contender for DNP practice should include primary care.

Practice Focus

A recent report issued by the National Governors Association (NGA; 2012) proposed that the passage of the Patient Protection and Affordable Care Act would be an important influence on the demand for primary care and the shortage of primary care providers. As a potential solution to the shortage of primary care providers, the NGA reviewed the literature on the quality and safety of NP practice and variation in regulations governing scope of practice across states. The authors concluded that "nurse practitioners are well qualified to deliver certain elements of primary care" and that ". . . states might consider changing scope of practice restrictions and assuring adequate reimbursement of their services" (p. 10). While this represents a qualified statement of support for NP practice; more important is the authors' opinion that NP expansion into primary care would increase access to health care.

A less timid approach to the shortage of primary care providers was taken by a multidisciplinary group convened by the Josiah Macy, Jr. Foundation in 2010. The conclusions and recommendations from the conference report represent many complexities in approaching the delivery of primary care, including the education and utilization of providers. The report, *Who Will Provide Primary Care and How Will They Be Trained?* (Culliton & Russell, 2010), recommended:

> Coupled with efforts to increase the number of physicians, nurse practitioners and physician assistants in primary care, state and national legal, regulatory, and reimbursement policies should be changed to remove barriers that make it difficult for nurse practitioners and physician assistants to serve as primary care providers and leaders of patient-centered medical homes or other models of primary care delivery. All primary care providers should be held accountable for the quality and efficiency of care as measured by patient outcomes. (p. 18)

Expansion of NPs into primary care, however, is not without its detractors. A recent study published in the *The New England Journal of Medicine* (Donelan,

DesRoches, Dittus, & Buerhaus, 2013) surveyed physicians and NPs in primary care to investigate attitudes about NP scope of practice, expansion of NPs into primary care, quality of NP practice, and equality of payment for similar services provided. Attitudes were mixed, but it is evident that physicians and NPs did not agree on roles in the delivery of primary care. Equal pay was the area of greatest disagreement among the two groups.

The bulk of the literature related to NP scope of practice and access to care supports the expansion of the NP role in primary care. Although the role and expertise of the DNP-prepared nurse remains somewhat broadly defined, there is no doubt that NPs are a significant feature in the future of primary care. An example of one particular practice focus for NPs, the comprehensive care specialty DNP developed by Columbia University School of Nursing, is useful for framing a discussion of the NP specialty in primary care.

Comprehensive Primary Care

Columbia University School of Nursing has a long tradition of advanced practice nursing education at the master's and DNP level. Following the guidance of the AACN, the curriculum is undergoing a transformation in order to educate all advanced practice nurses at the DNP level with a phase out of master's preparation for the advanced practice role. The preparation for Columbia's advanced practice nurse is the comprehensive care specialty. This can be best described as an advanced practice nurse with a comprehensive specialty focus who can "demonstrate expertise in the provision, coordination, and direction of comprehensive care to patients, including those who present in healthy states and over time" (Columbia University School of Nursing [CUSN], 2012a).

The planned DNP curriculum will be comprised of a 3-year course of study that begins with three semesters of comprehensive care content including chronic illness, informatics, and genetics; four semesters of specialty content; and two semesters in a clinical residency and completion of a portfolio project. The specialty content beginning in the third semester prepares the DNP graduate to qualify as a nurse midwife, nurse anesthetist, family practitioner, pediatric practitioner, adult/geriatric practitioner, psychiatric/mental health practitioner, or acute care practitioner (CUSN, 2012b).

The content of the comprehensive care DNP specialty incorporates the competencies for comprehensive care. These competencies were first developed in 2010 (Honig & Smolowitz, 2010) and revised in 2011. The competencies include four content domains and 19 competencies. Within Domain 1, Comprehensive Clinical Care, are six competencies, including evaluation of patient needs; evaluation of health risk; formulation of differential diagnoses; appraisal of acuity; evaluation, care, and discharge plan with acute care; and comprehensive care in a subacute setting. Domain 2, Interdisciplinary and Patient-Centered Commination, contains four competencies, including collaborative interdisciplinary network for referral and consultation; managing chronic illness, including care transitions; translation of health information and incorporating shared decision making with the patient; and the facilitation of palliative care and end-of-life care (CUSN, 2011).

Domain 3, Systems and Context of Care, contains four competencies, including culturally sensitive and individualized interventions; evaluation of gaps in care, including knowledge of the organization and financing of health care systems; principles of legal and ethical decision making; and integrating principles of business, finance, economics, and health policy in designing population-based initiatives. The final domain, Building and Using Evidence for Best Clinical Practices and Scholarship, contains five competencies, including synthesize and analyze evidence; evaluate quality of care; critically appraise and synthesize research findings; assess and critically appraise clinical scholarship; and utilize informatics tools to identify best practices (CUSN, 2011).

The vision expressed by the faculty at Columbia University School of Nursing is that advanced practice at the doctoral level ought to achieve significant outcomes in revolutionizing the provision of comprehensive primary care across the lifespan in all settings, particularly for populations living with chronic illness and populations vulnerable to poor health status because of compromising determinants of health. To achieve these aims, education must focus on prevention and health protection, systems of care, complex diagnosis and management of illness, and advocacy for health-promoting environments (CUSN, 2012b).

Assuring the Quality of DNP Practice

Most professionals, particularly those within the health field, utilize a standardized system of licensure, accreditation, certification, and education to assure quality. While we are acutely aware that assuring quality is a tricky business, the health professions have established fairly complex requirements at the provider, organization, and educational levels to achieve safe and effective outcomes. Long ago nursing adopted licensure as entry into the profession.

With the addition of advanced clinical roles and higher complexity in education and health care, nursing added the requirements of accreditation of education programs, certification to recognize the expertise and achievement of standards of practice, and formal and standardized educational programs that grant degrees or postgraduate certificates. This regulatory model for nursing (LACE: licensing, accreditation, certification, education) has become the norm for advanced practice registered nurses (Nurse Practitioner Joint Dialogue Group Report, 2008). The LACE document outlines the definition of the advanced practice nurse, titling for the recognized roles (clinical nurse specialist, certified registered nurse anesthetist, certified nurse–midwife, and certified NP), and broadly defined educational benchmarks. Although the LACE document went a long way in laying the groundwork for a system of recognition and assurance of quality and standards, the actual recognition of each component of LACE has many variations. Numerous specialty organizations credential nursing specialty practice and each state has jurisdiction over nursing licensure.

Specialty titles are still not recognized equally across the United States. Educational accreditation has numerous tiers and layers of accreditation, with separate accrediting bodies for programs and specialties. At the end of the day, the question remains: Does this all make a difference in achieving quality outcomes for the consumer?

This question is at the heart of a new IOM Standing Committee: *Standing Committee on Credentialing Research in Nursing*. The committee members represent many perspectives on credentialing and many different disciplines. The primary task of the standing committee is to engage in dialogue and seek information on emerging priorities for nursing credentialing research; research methodologies and measures relevant to nursing credentialing research; the impact of individual and organizational credentialing in nursing on improving health care performance, quality, and outcomes; and strategic planning for moving the field of credentialing research forward (IOM, 2013). It remains to be seen whether research will show that credentialing for nursing, without a doubt, leads to superior outcomes for those we serve. We take this for granted, but the research is not conclusive. This IOM Standing Committee will seek to understand this dilemma in more depth.

Meanwhile, another challenge presents itself: Do the licensing and credentialing requirements for master's-prepared advanced practice registered nurses apply to those with a practice doctorate? Should there be additional or different certification requirements that attest to the competencies for DNP education? Schools of nursing are accredited for meeting the *Essentials* of DNP education, but what about the individual practitioner?

The American Board of Comprehensive Care Certification Exam

This challenge prompted the 2007 founding of the American Board of Comprehensive Care (ABCC). This board is the certifying organization for doctoral-level advanced practice nurses in the comprehensive care specialty. The ABCC teamed with the National Board of Medical Examiners to develop and administer a certification exam that, upon passage, awards the Diplomat of Comprehensive Care (DCC) designation. The exam measures the same set of competencies administered to physicians as the final component of their licensure exam (Step 3 of the United States Medical Licensing Examination). While the exam is not required for DNP practice, the ABCC believes that successful passage of this exam recognizes the specialized role of the practice doctorate for clinicians and may enable the differentiation of practice across educational preparation and DNP roles. The exam is only offered to DNP graduates who hold national certification as an advanced practice registered nurse (CUSN, 2012a).

The Scholarship of DNP Practice

This introductory chapter outlining the emergence and impact of DNP education would not be complete without a comment on contributions to scholarship by those who hold the degree and practice in one of the DNP roles. The role of the DNP in scholarship stimulated significant discussion about how or whether to differentiate scholarship and research between the DNP and PhD. It seems to me that a clear case has been made through the *Essentials* of DNP education that the DNP is well suited for scholarship in the application of evidence to practice, the clinical innovation required to enhance quality outcomes within practice settings, and to examine variation in effectiveness across approaches to care and recommend those that achieve higher value to patients and populations.

According to *The Essentials of Doctoral Education for Advanced Nursing Practice* (2006), the DNP graduate takes a "practice application-oriented" (p. 3) approach to scholarship. However, many PhD-prepared scientists also explore applications of science to problems in practice. Language from the *Essentials* document states that the DNP graduate will "develop and evaluate new practice approaches based on nursing theories and theories from other disciplines" and will "develop and evaluate care delivery approaches that meet current and future needs of patient populations based on scientific findings in nursing and other clinical sciences, as well as organization, political, and economic sciences" (p. 10). These are certainly areas for scholarship but may not necessitate the development of new knowledge. A practical approach to gaining understanding of the field of DNP scholarship was to review publications in the *Clinical Scholars Review: The Journal of Doctoral Nursing Practice.*

Several themes emerged from a review of the published literature in this journal. First, a good portion of the literature is descriptive of the DNP degree, DNP certification, and challenges faced in practice and defining the role. For example, Starck and Woolbert (2010) argued that one method of distinguishing the clinical practice DNP role from the nondirect care role was through distinct certification such as the DNP Comprehensive Care Certification. Through a certification process, common competencies of DNP practice could be demonstrated. A second set of themes was related to DNP education.

Wright, Scherb, and Forsyth (2011) reviewed the literature on education using online strategies, identified gaps in the literature, and developed a tool for evaluating online student-based discussion as part of their learning environment. Evidence for practice was the third major theme. Some of the articles are descriptive of how evidence-based practice knowledge is developed in DNP education, and several other examples were informative as examples of scholarship undertaken for practice-related questions. McCauley (2012) studied the effect of introducing an evidence-based approach to reducing central line infections in an intensive care unit. A specific theoretical model for adaptation of new guidelines was used. The results of this study showed a decrease in infections. The nurses' attitudes about using guidelines and whether guidelines improve nursing knowledge were also examined. Another good example of DNP scholarship is a study by Amendolia (2011) that reports on an integrative review of the literature to understand feeding intolerance among preterm infants. The purpose of the study was to provide a review of the state of the science in this particular area of practice.

If DNP programs focus on scholarship that enhances the utilization of evidence-based practice and quality management within practice settings, we can be confident that our graduates will combine practice expertise with knowledge of clinical innovation for enhanced patient and population health outcomes. In a way, the capstone portion of DNP education was designed to test this assumption. Do DNP students gain methodological skills that enhance inquiry related to the application of evidence to practice? Are they able to interpret and critique the literature so they are prepared to apply innovation in the practice settings and measure the outcomes? Certainly from what we see in the literature so far, I am optimistic that this is so.

FROM EVOLUTION TO REVOLUTION

Considering the slow uptake of most innovation in health care, it is somewhat revolutionary that this relatively new degree and practice role have sustained a growth trend. Many of us in the field of education are engaged in transformation of one type or another to embrace the early vision of the pioneers who conceptualized this new role. We are collaborating with practice leaders to evaluate the impact of the role on patient outcomes and health systems. While we may disagree and debate about the future of the role, we agree that health care and society need nurses who are able to manage complexity, lead change, and create innovation. We believe this is an important approach to solving the shortage of primary care providers, to enhance the quality and value of health systems, and to meet the interest and passion of nurses who want to contribute to health care in an advanced role in an arena different than but in partnership with research colleagues.

To assure that DNP-prepared nurses continue to revolutionize the way care is provided and evaluated, we in academic institutions must foster ongoing assurance that the role maintains its prominence as a practice doctorate. We must resist the temptation to blur the distinctions between the practice and research doctorates. At the same time we must take care to establish pathways to recognition and promotion for DNP faculty and to incentivize collaboration among practice and research faculty in academia and through our DNP- and PhD-prepared health system partners. The evolution of nursing as a profession with a distinct practice and research frame has no doubt been slow—painfully so to many of us. The emergence of this new role is a clear signal to society that nursing is not finished evolving yet; not by a long shot!

REFERENCES

Amendolia, B. (2011). An integrative review of feeding intolerance in preterm infants: State of the science. *Clinical Scholars Review, 4*(2), 82–90.

American Association of Colleges of Nursing. (2004). *AACN position statement on the practice doctorate in nursing.* Retrieved from http://www.aacn.nche.edu/DNP/pdf/DNP.pdf

American Association of Colleges of Nursing. (2006). *The essentials of doctoral education for advanced nursing practice.* Retrieved from http://www.aacn.nche.edu/education-resources/essential-series

American Association of Colleges of Nursing. (2013, April). *DNP fact sheet.* Retrieved from http://www.aacn.nche.edu/media-relations/fact-sheets/dnp

Centers for Medicare & Medicaid Services. (2009). *Roadmap for implementing value driven healthcare in the traditional Medicare fee-for-service program.* Retrieved from http://www.cms.gov/Medicare/Quality-Initiatives-Patient-Assessment-Instruments/QualityInitiativesGenInfo/Downloads/VBPRoadmap_OEA_1-16_508.pdf

Centers for Medicare & Medicaid Services. (2013, April 17). *Medicare FFS physician feedback program/value-based payment modifier.* Retrieved from http://www.cms.gov/Medicare/Medicare-Fee-for-Service-Payment/PhysicianFeedbackProgram

Columbia University School of Nursing. (2011). *DNP competencies for comprehensive care.* Retrieved from http://www.cumc.columbia.edu/nursing/academics/pdf/DNPCompetencies2011%282%29.pdf

Columbia University School of Nursing. (2012a). *The American board of comprehensive care.* Retrieved from http://www.cumc.columbia.edu/nursing/dnpcert/index.shtml

Columbia University School of Nursing. (2012b). *Doctor of nursing practice (DNP): Post baccalaureate and post master's.* Retrieved from http://www.cumc.columbia.edu/nursing/academics/dnp.php

Cronenwett, L., Dracup, K., Grey, M., McCauley, L., Meleis, A., & Salmon, M. (2011). The doctor of nursing practice: A national workforce perspective. *Nursing Outlook, 59*(1), 9–17. doi:10.1016/j.outlook.2010.11.003

Culliton, B. J., & Russell, S. (Eds.). (2010). *Who will provide primary care and how will they be trained?* [Conference proceedings]. Durham, NC: Josiah Macy, Jr. Foundation.

Donelan, K., DesRoches, C. M., Dittus, R. S., & Buerhaus, P. (2013). Perspectives of physicians and nurse practitioners on primary care practice. *The New England Journal of Medicine, 368*(20), 1898–1906. doi:10.1056/NEJMsa1212938

Dunbar-Jacob, J., Nativio, D. G., & Khalil, H. (2013). Impact of doctor of nursing practice education in shaping health care systems for the future. *Journal of Nursing Education, 52*(8), 423–427. doi:10.3928/01484834-20130719-03

Honig, J., & Smolowitz, J. (2010). Development of DNP competencies in comprehensive care. In J. Smolowitz, J. Honig, & C. Reinisch (Eds.), *Writing DNP clinical case narratives: Demonstrating and evaluating competency in comprehensive care* (pp.15–26). New York, NY: Springer Publishing Company.

Institute of Medicine. (1999). *To err is human: Building a safer health system.* Washington, DC: National Academies Press. Retrieved from http://www.iom.edu/Reports/1999/to-err-is-human-building-a-safer-health-system.aspx

Institute of Medicine. (2001). *Crossing the quality chasm: A new health system for the 21st century.* Washington, DC: The National Academies Press. Retrieved from http://www.iom.edu/Reports/2001/Crossing-the-Quality-Chasm-A-New-Health-System-for-the-21st-Century.aspx

Institute of Medicine. (2003). *Health professions education: A bridge to quality.* Washington, DC: National Academies Press. Retrieved from http://www.iom.edu/Reports/2003/health-professions-education-a-bridge-to-quality.aspx

Institute of Medicine. (2010). *The future of nursing: Leading change, advancing health.* Washington, DC: The National Academies Press. Retrieved from http://www.iom.edu/Reports/2010/The-future-of-nursing-leading-change-advancing-health.aspx

Institute of Medicine. (2013, November 15). *Standing Committee on Credentialing Research in Nursing.* Retrieved from http://www.iom.edu/activities/workforce/nursingcredentialing.aspx

McCauley, P. (2012). Evidence-based clinical guidelines and their impact on prevention of catheter-related bloodstream infections. *Clinical Scholars Review, 5*(1), 18–30.

National Committee for Quality Assurance. (n.d.). *The essential guide to health care quality.* Retrieved from http://www.ncqa.org/Portals/0/Publications/Resource%20Library/NCQA_Primer_web.pdf

National Council of State Boards of Nursing. (2008). *Consensus model for nurse practitio-ner regulation: Licensure, accreditation, certification & education* (Nurse Practitioner Joint Dialogue Group Report). Retrieved from https://www.ncsbn.org/4213.htm

National Governors Association. (2012). *The role of nurse practitioners in meeting increas-ing demand for primary care*. Retrieved from NGA Center for Best Practices website: http://www.nga.org/cms/home/nga-center-for-best-practices/center-publications/page-health-publications/col2-content/main-content-list/the-role-of-nurse-practitioners.html

National Quality Forum. (2013). *Measurement evaluation criteria*. Retrieved from http://www.qualityforum.org/docs/measure_evaluation_criteria.aspx

Newhouse, R. P., Stanik-Hutt, J., White, K. M., Johantgen, M., Bass, E. B., Zangaro, G., . . . Weiner, J. P. (2011). NP outcomes 1990–2008: A systematic review. *Nursing Eco-nomic$*, *37*(5), 230–251.

Starck, P. L., & Woolbert, L. (2010). DNP comprehensive care certification: What are the issues? *Clinical Scholars Review*, *3*(2), 59–63.

United States Department of Health and Human Services. (2010). *Affordable Care and Reconciliation Act*. Retrieved from HHS.gov/HealthCare website: http://www.hhs.gov/healthcare/rights/law/index.html

Wright, T. L., Scherb, C. A., & Forsyth, D. M. (2011). A rubric for evaluating online discussion contributions of graduate nursing students. *Clinical Scholars Review*, *4*(1), 5–14.

2

BSN to DNP: The Journey to Exemplary Capstone Projects

Judith A. Kaufmann

Robert Morris University (RMU) in Pittsburgh, Pennsylvania, was one of the initial bachelor's in science of nursing (BSN) to doctor of nursing (DNP) programs established in the United States. The program was started in 2007 and was among the first BSN-DNP programs accredited by the Commission on Collegiate Nursing Education (CCNE) in 2010.

This chapter describes the development of the RMU DNP program and the evolution of the DNP capstone as the program progressed.

Dr. Kaufmann highlights exemplary DNP capstones that demonstrate the growth of the students as they begin the program as BSNs and emerge as doctorally prepared advanced practice registered nurses with leadership and translational research skills.

Joyce M. Knestrick, Editor

This chapter addresses issues related to the development of the bachelor's in science of nursing to doctor of nursing (BSN-DNP) capstone curriculum, including translation of research into practice and use of evidence in clinical capstone projects by nurse practitioner (NP) students at Robert Morris University (RMU). RMU is a small, private university that opened the BSN-DNP program in 2007, and was among the first BSN-DNP programs accredited by the Commission on Collegiate Nursing Education (CCNE) in 2010. As one of the pioneers in this new degree, RMU has valuable lessons learned to share.

THE NATIONAL MOVEMENT TOWARD BSN TO DNP

In 2004, the American Association of Colleges of Nursing (AACN) voted to endorse the *Position Statement on the Practice Doctorate in Nursing.* This document can be retrieved from http://www.aacn.nche.edu/DNP/DNPPositionStatement .htm. Since then, there has been rapid movement in the development of DNP programs across the United States. To date, most of the programs have been at the postmaster's of science in nursing (MSN) level. Once the target date of 2015 was set as a goal for the transition of nurse practitioner (NP) programs to the DNP level for entry to advanced practice, there has also been progression in development of BSN-DNP programs.

At the time of this writing, there are 116 accredited post-master's DNP programs and 115 post baccalaureate programs (AACN, 2013). While there are variations in the curriculum designs, all the programs are focused on outcomes consistent with producing advanced practice registered nurses (APRNs), who will assume or maintain clinical practice roles and function at the highest level consistent with their academic preparation (Institute of Medicine [IOM], 2010). Now that the Patient Protection and Affordable Care Act is implemented (United States Department of Health and Human Services [USDHHS], 2010), NPs are at the forefront of primary care. NPs will be cost-effective care providers in both acute and long-term care settings (American Academy of Nursing [AAN], 2010).

Given the rapid changes in the health care system, the impending policies, and federally subsidized health care plan mandates, NP education programs must respond. Stakeholders include practitioners, hospitals, patients, physicians, payers, and government oversight agencies. The nation is watching as NPs move toward autonomous practice and play increasingly visible roles within health care systems.

Never has it been more crucial to the nursing profession than now for academically well-prepared NPs to step into positions of increased responsibility, both professionally and legally. Based on the assumption that education makes a difference in clinical practice, as well as the national call for an increased number of doctoral-prepared nurses (IOM, 2010), there has been a rush to establish accredited BSN-DNP programs with well-defined benchmarks. Never has an academic degree generated such controversy, curiosity, skepticism, and excitement both within and outside of the discipline of nursing.

The Essentials of Doctoral Education for Advanced Nursing Practice (AACN, 2006) calls for assurance of high-quality clinical competencies in direct patient care and translation of research into practice. The *Essentials* describe the need to understand and address leadership, system change, and improvement in health care delivery through interdisciplinary teamwork. Recruiting practicing APRNs into DNP programs is a short-term response to the IOM recommendations. The postmaster's programs are relatively short, as the number of credits required for a clinical doctorate is predicated on a high number of credits required in MSN-level education (ranging from 45 to 55 credits). Most post-master's programs can be completed within 2 years or less, with an average length of 21 months, as compared to an average length of 40 months for a BSN-DNP program.

The time frame for preparing NPs at the doctoral level poses significant concerns, with the demand for NPs increasing while the pool of postmaster's practicing NPs and primary care physicians cannot fill the gap. While experienced NPs seeking postmaster's DNP degrees have a wealth of experience and knowledge, BSN-DNP students enter programs with minimal understanding of the demands of time, money, responsibility, and expectation in the NP role.

Educators must have clear expectations about the realities of rigorous BSN-DNP programs and be cognizant of the potential for rapid student (and faculty) burn-out associated with the 1,000 clinical hours, expanded course content, and final capstone projects. BSN-DNP students bring minimal clinical experience to an advanced practice role from which to evaluate and translate current evidence into capstone projects.

Despite differences inherent in the two tracks culminating in a DNP degree (BSN-DNP and postmaster's DNP), the expected competencies are the same (AACN, 2006). Outcomes for DNP capstones place less emphasis on generation of theory and new knowledge and more emphasis on translation of research into grounded clinical practice in actual patient settings. Secondary analysis of existing data is also recommended as a basis for ongoing improvement in delivery of patient care. Helping students to refine and define a project that is realistic and pertinent to the issues facing health care systems, patients, and providers, and at the appropriate level of research skills, is often difficult.

AN EXEMPLAR OF BSN-DNP PROGRAM DEVELOPMENT

The development of the BSN-DNP curriculum at the RMU School of Nursing occurred in lieu of an MSN-level NP program. The BSN-DNP program was designed within 3 years of opening an undergraduate BSN program. Since there was no existing MSN-NP program at the university, the decision was made to construct a DNP curriculum from the onset, incorporating the DNP *Essentials* at the inception rather than transitioning from an existing MSN-NP program. Early in the planning process, the graduate faculty established benchmarks that would guide program evaluation as a basis for ongoing quality improvement (QI) and program revision. These benchmarks included:

- CCNE accreditation
- Documentation of national certification pass rates
- Annual online student surveys and focus group feedback
- Student retention rates
- Small grant funding
- Published manuscripts in peer-reviewed journals
- Local, regional, and national presentations
- Leadership and/or advisory positions in professional organizations or health systems
- Ongoing postgraduation scholarly clinical projects
- Job placement/advancement/satisfaction

The curriculum was designed to integrate DNP competencies beginning in the first semester. Students enter the program as a cohort each fall. The program begins with an applied statistics course, preparing students to critically assess data-based publications with a basic understanding of health care research statistics. Subsequent clinical management courses, including the three Ps (pathophysiology, physical assessment and diagnosis, and pharmacology) are weighted heavily with assignments that require clinical decisions based on high-quality evidence. In Year 2, students are introduced to the relationship between direct patient care and population health concepts in health promotion, clinical prevention, and epidemiology. Basic biostatistics are presented within the context of public health implications and routine clinical care decisions. The focus is on the transference of evidence into patient care, emphasizing the NP role as clinician with primary responsibility for safe and competent patient care. A model for curriculum design is seen in Figure 2.1.

While there may be a tendency to gravitate toward nurse researcher roles and to subordinate clinical practice, it is critical that the identity of the DNP is framed within clinical competency and regarded as separate but equal with a research doctorate.

Research and Clinical Translation

An example of the need to clearly define clinical translation of research occurred recently. A third-year BSN-DNP student was interested in working with a non–university-affiliated hospital that had contacted the University requesting an external evaluation of their readmission assessment screening tool. As with all hospitals, readmission rates would soon be posing a financial threat. The hospital had existing data on screening scores and admission rates, which, to date, had not been analyzed for predictive value. The hospital had created its own screening tool as opposed to using a standardized tool because

FIGURE 2.1 *Integration of NP and DNP Competencies Into Curriculum*

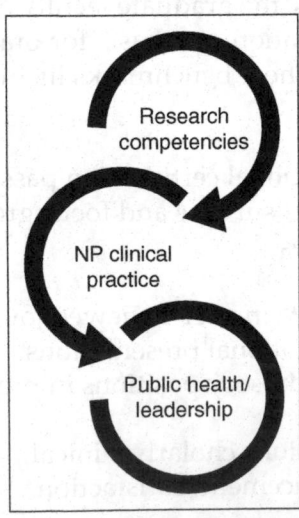

the hospital representatives considered the 60% to 70% accuracy of existing tools unacceptable.

Upon a thorough search of the literature, the BSN-DNP student found a screening tool with reported 85% accuracy and suggested the use of this tool. Rather than review and analyze existing data, she wanted to implement a new protocol and collect prospective data, a much more exciting project from her perspective. As expected, it became apparent that the goals of the institution were not consistent with the student's goals. In subsequent meetings, she became frustrated when the hospital's QI committee rejected the implementation of the tool.

The capstone advisor reminded the student that translational research involves integrating research into practice, working within systems to improve quality, and evaluating existing initiatives prior to implementing new initiatives. In other words, "How did she know if the present screening tool was 'broken' before she would try to fix it?"

To further make a case for analysis of existing data, the faculty helped the student to understand that a prospective study would take at least 2 to 3 years for a valid comparison of readmission screening tools. In addition, she would meet barriers in the form of the institutional IRB, given the institution's reluctance to change present protocols without evidence to suggest that the current system was not working. Therefore, her very enthusiastic project would not be feasible given academic and institutional time constraints. The student was in a position to potentially assume future leadership and change a system if she could provide outcomes data on current practice. This evolution of a capstone project illustrates just one of the issues that can arise in clarifying the difference between research and clinical translation with the BSN-DNP student.

Program Length

Students entering BSN-DNP programs face three very formidable challenges: the length of the program; the increased tuition costs; and the expanded curriculum that demands content focused on individual patient care, translational research, population health, and organizational systems. The number of credits required for the BSN-DNP program may range from 80 to 86 credits, with 1,000 direct contact clinical hours over a 3- to 4-year period. The second challenge is the need for the student to graduate and enter the NP workforce in a timely manner in order to meet the high demand for high-level direct care providers. The time span between the "Three Ps" and the management courses and capstone project may pose a potential threat to successful passage of the certification exam. Other barriers include additional tuition costs, stress, and the potential for first-time failure on certification exams.

To address these issues, RMU integrates the capstone project into the curriculum beginning in the second year of the program, so that the DNP Essentials are concurrent with the clinical NP competencies rather than in a tiered format where DNP-specific courses and the capstone project are deferred to the last year. A capstone timeline outlines the progression of the capstone throughout the curriculum (Table 2.1).

TABLE 2.1 **BSN-DNP Timeline for a Capstone Project**

Semester	Course	Capstone Competency	Responsibility

Fall Year 2	Research and Theory	1. Identify potential area of interest
		2. Conduct a preliminary literature review
		3. Consider type of project
		   a. _____program evaluation
		   b. _____qualitative project (with special permission)
		   c. _____quantitative project
		   d. _____systems improvement
			Course instructor

Summer Year 2	Integrating Research Into Practice	1. Complete written literature review
		2. Submit draft of project proposal
		  • To include:
		   a. Significance and background for project
		   b. Specific aim and projected outcomes for project
		   c. Methodology
		     i. ____design of project
		     ii. ____site for project
		     iii. ____sample or participants
		September: DNP faculty and course instructors will meet to assign tentative capstone advisees
		3. One-page project summary to be sent to advisor: STUDENT responsibility
			Course instructor/s
			
			Course instructors and DNP faculty
			Capstone advisor

Spring Year 3	EBP and Advanced Nursing Roles	1. PowerPoint Overview for faculty
		2. Submit IRB Proposal
		
		   a. Identify measurement tool (based on literature/published instruments)
		   b. Determine outcomes analysis plan
		
		IRB to be submitted by last day of spring semester
			Capstone advisor and course instructors
			Course instructor and capstone advisor
			Course instructor, advisor, and statistician
			Capstone advisor

(continued)

TABLE 2.1 BSN-DNP Timeline for a Capstone Project (continued)

Semester	Course	Capstone Competency	Responsibility
Summer Year 3	EBP and Information Systems	1. Implement project and collect data 2. Enter data into spreadsheet (Excel or database of choice) 3. Begin analysis of data (December–January)	Course instructor, capstone advisor, and statistician
Spring Year 4	Applying EBP in Health Care Settings	1. Identify potential journal for publication submission 2. Write abstract for professional presentation 3. Complete manuscript for publication adhering to publication guidelines 4. Complete PowerPoint presentation	9620 course instructor and capstone advisor Capstone advisor must sign final approval of capstone project and PowerPoint presentation prior to the presentation

DNP, doctor of nursing practice; EBP, evidence-based practice; IRB, institutional review board.

Adherence to this timeline allows for input from a number of faculty, thus replacing the need for a traditional committee and minimizing faculty workload. By project completion, students have had the benefit of approaching the clinical problem from a number of perspectives, with at least three additional faculty in collaboration with their capstone advisor and a statistical consultant.

Students are encouraged to conduct their projects at their clinical sites. This approach allows students to appreciate the importance of implementing evidence-based management and evaluating patient outcomes as part of daily clinical practice. This approach also saves time, as it incorporates the capstone project into the expanded clinical hours. The following illustrates the integration of clinical practice and capstone project by a psychiatric mental health NP student.

As a result of this project, the NP student was offered a full-time position upon graduation, not only to provide direct NP care, but to assume responsibilities for further evaluation of patient outcomes and QI practice initiatives.

Clinical Sites and DNP Project Development

Another challenge encountered by the BSN-DNP students that may not be a problem with practicing APRNs in postmaster's DNP programs is the need for

FIGURE 2.2 *Exemplar of a Capstone Project Integrated Into Clinical Hours*

Evaluating Diagnostic Accuracy of Child and Adolescent Attention Deficit Hyperactivity Disorder as Diagnosed in Primary Care Versus Psychiatry Specialty: A Case for Integration

Abstract

PURPOSE: The purpose of this project was to examine the rate of attention deficit hyperactivity disorder (ADHD) diagnoses among children and adolescents when a structured interview, the Mini-International Neuropsychiatric Interview–Kid Version (MINI-KID), is administered versus the diagnosis made in the primary care setting, commonly with the use of screening instruments. Accurate diagnosis is imperative to assist in prompt and accurate pharmacological and psychosocial intervention, as inaccurate diagnosis can lead to detrimental effects of improper medication prescription.

AIM/DESIGN: This study used a single-group correlational design evaluating 10 subjects diagnosed with ADHD in a primary care setting who were then referred to child and adolescent psychiatry. The psychiatry consult included the administration of the MINI-KID by the doctor of nursing practice (DNP)/Family Psychiatric Mental Health Nurse Practitioner (FPMHNP) candidate or a master's degree-prepared mental health therapist. The diagnoses formulated by primary care prior to referral and by the MINI-KID were compared with the results of the diagnostic interview conducted by the board-certified child and adolescent psychiatrist.

METHODS: Both male and female subjects ages 7 to 15 were recruited from patients referred to the outpatient psychiatry office of Neurobehavioral Medicine Consultants. Data collected included the psychiatric diagnosis made by the primary care provider (PCP) and any subsequently prescribed psychotropic medications; the psychiatric diagnosis determined with use of the MINI-KID; the psychiatric diagnosis made by the psychiatrist and any subsequently prescribed psychotropic medications; and demographic data of all subjects.

RESULTS: The results of this study revealed at least an 80% diagnostic concordance between the MINI-KID and the child and adolescent psychiatrist for ADHD, mood disorders, and obsessive-compulsive disorder (OCD). Additionally, there is 80% agreement in the diagnosis of ADHD by the PCP and the psychiatrist; however, the psychiatrist diagnosed a comorbid mood disorder in 50% of the study participants.

CONCLUSION: Both the challenges and benefits of integrated primary and psychiatric care are well described in the current body of literature. This pilot study's results indicated that PCPs adeptly diagnose and treat ADHD in children and adolescents, but often comorbid psychiatric conditions, in particular mood disorders, are also present. Specialized psychiatric services are necessary to accurately identify and treat these often complex clinical presentations.

clinical sites for the capstone project. Most postmaster's DNP students enter programs with a general idea of a question or clinical initiative they would like to address in their capstone work, and it is the job of the program to equip these students with evidence-based tools as a foundation for their projects. The sites for their projects and potential clinical collaborators may not be an issue.

At the BSN-DNP level, students have been predominantly practicing at staff nurse levels and most have not been actively involved in research at their clinical facilities. The main question for BSN-DNP faculty is how to facilitate capstone projects that are pertinent to NP practice for students who have not yet attained reputations within their facilities. The dilemma is establishing clinical experiences and sites that foster DNP capstone project development.

One possible solution is to establish a symbiotic relationship between the academic and the clinical facility. What resources can the university provide for private hospitals to assist them in providing evidence of patient care outcomes? What problems have community hospitals identified that can be translated into academic capstone projects for BSN-DNP students? The answer lies in forming collaborative relationships between hospital administrators, QI officers, and DNP faculty.

The collaborative model that has proven efficacious at RMU is to designate one faculty person as the *point person* for potential collaboration with outside health care facilities. Assignment of one contact from each clinical facility further facilitates this relationship. Facilities often have mounds of data that have not been analyzed. This data can be valuable for BSN-DNP students learning to search current literature, interpret statistics, and perform secondary analysis. These data exist as part of mandated performance measures that are now being tied to reimbursement (National Committee for Quality Assurance [NCQA], 2005).

In order to remain financially viable, hospitals are mandated to provide evidence of patient outcomes for third-party payers. One example of a BSN-DNP student capstone project that demonstrates collaboration between the BSN-DNP program and a non–university-affiliated hospital system follows.

These exemplar capstone projects (Figures 2.2 and 2.3) demonstrate the value of building DNP scholarly projects around real-world problems encountered in the clinical setting. The National Organization of Nurse Practitioner Faculties (NONPF) requires the attainment of NP competencies within the educational program (NONPF, 2012). The RMU capstone project model demonstrates that BSN-DNP students can design capstone projects while attaining these competencies.

Translational Research

The goal of the BSN-DNP program is to prepare competent direct-care providers. NPs are in demand because they provide high-quality care and are economically feasible to health care systems, generating income for practices and hospitals. Generally, the expanded clinical hours prepare the BSN-DNP student to enter the job market with confidence and a short learning curve.

Added value is the ability to apply evidence-based concepts to patient outcomes and to be a part of a research team that is typically led by a PhD-prepared

FIGURE 2.3 *Exemplar of a Hospital–Capstone Project Collaboration*

Patient and Hospital-Based Risk Factors and the Occurrence of Venous Thromboembolic Events Following Total Hip or Knee Replacement: A Correlational Study

Abstract

BACKGROUND: Venous thromboembolism (VTE) is a common, often fatal, and costly injury that complicates major orthopedic surgery and can lead to increases in medical costs, lengths of hospital stay, and increased morbidity and mortality. While much research has been done on the topic and thromboprophylactic guidelines have been standardized, VTE is still the most common cause of hospital readmission and death following total joint replacement.

SPECIFIC AIM: The overall aim of this study was to identify patient and practice variables related to venous thromboembolic events within 30 days status post elective total hip or knee replacement.

METHODS: This correlational study was conducted in collaboration with a multidisciplinary team from a suburban Pittsburgh hospital. A two-group correlational retrospective design was used to identify significant factors related to postoperative VTEs following total joint replacement over a period of 30 months. The data were analyzed using a univariate, binary logistic regression with multiple predictors.

POPULATION: Patient population included all patients who underwent total hip or total knee replacement between August 2008 and February 2011 and subsequently developed a VTE within 30 days of surgery. Matching patients based on demographic data identified a control group. This group included joint replacement patients who did not develop VTE. As per IRB committee requests, a 1:3 case-to-control ratio was utilized. A total of 160 patients undergoing total hip or knee replacement at a suburban Pittsburgh hospital were included in the study. Forty of these patients were diagnosed with a VTE within 30 days of their joint replacement. A control group was identified by matching demographic data and included 120 patients who did not experience VTE complications.

RESULTS: The development of venous thromboemboli following total hip or knee replacement cannot be attributed to a single root cause. While the cause of VTE is multifactorial, it can be predicted with some accuracy in patients with multiple risk factors. While some of these risk factors are nonmodifiable, others are modifiable and can be eliminated or amended to reduce a patient's relative risk of developing VTE following major orthopedic surgery. These modifiable patient risk factors include current smoking status and BMI. Other risk factors that are hospital based and controllable can also be targeted to improve patient outcomes, such as limiting tourniquet time, encouraging patient ambulation on surgical day, prescribing physical therapy, ordering mechanical prophylaxis, and utilizing standardized guidelines regarding VTE chemoprophylaxis, and appear to reduce the incidence of VTE.

colleague. Based on the previously stated assumptions, DNP-prepared nurses should not be expected to lead research teams or independently design high-level research studies. Nor are they expected to generate new evidence based on clinical trials or meta-analysis studies. These limitations do not imply that DNP nurses assume subordinate roles on the research team. Rather, they can be expected to translate research into clinical care settings, especially those where patients have multiple comorbidities that might otherwise exclude them from controlled experimental trials. DNP nurses must be able to communicate with PhD researchers using research terms and concepts with a solid understanding of statistical principles and underlying assumptions.

As such, capstone projects should be expected to be internally valid although rarely generalizable. Suggested clinical research designs appropriate to capstone projects include descriptive pre-/post-, correlational, case-control (ex post facto), cross-sectional, and program evaluation. All of these suggested designs can be useful for evaluating patient outcomes and/or QI initiatives.

Equally important is the fact that these research designs can be relatively inexpensive and uncomplicated, requiring basic statistics to evaluate outcomes. Examples of capstone topics and appropriate research designs are seen in Table 2.2.

There is limited time in the BSN-DNP program for more than one statistics course, given the magnitude of clinical hours and intensive specialty coursework required to meet NONPF competencies. The program at RMU integrates statistical skills into all evidence-based research classes and clinical specialty

TABLE 2.2 *Research Design and Capstone Topic*

Research Design	Capstone Topic	Statistical Options
Pre-/post	Clinical accuracy of identifying heart murmurs in nurse practitioner students before and after simulation	Descriptive statistics and paired *t*-tests
Cross-sectional	Clinicians' acceptance factors and perceived barriers to EHRs	Descriptive and correlational statistics
Correlational	Transmission of MRSA and room assignments	Correlational statistics
Case control (ex post facto)	Factors associated with infection in patients after total joint replacement	Relative risk Odds ratios ANOVA
Program evaluation	Development and use of educational DVD for patients diagnosed with CHF to decrease readmission rates	Formative: descriptive Summative: paired and independent samples *t*-test

ANOVA, analysis of variance; CHF, congestive heart failure; EHR, electronic health record; MRSA, methicillin-resistant *Staphylococcus aureus*.

FIGURE 2.4 *Course Objectives for Statistics in Health Care*

Understand and interpret quantitative data in data-based research articles

Determine appropriate statistical tests based on research questions and patient outcome goals

Interpret and present results of data analysis

Identify appropriate statistical tests based on underlying test assumptions

Address limitations of data based on sample and effect size, and power and characteristics of data

Identify appropriate indications for use of biostatistics

Identify components of data collection for tests and measures in the educational process

Use statistical analysis to evaluate quality of tests/measurements in the educational process

FIGURE 2.5 *Exemplar of Statistical Level in a DNP Capstone*

Does obesity impact in-hospital outcomes following primary percutaneous coronary intervention in patients with acute ST-elevation myocardial infarction?

Abstract

INTRODUCTION: Acute myocardial infarction is among the leading causes of mortality in the United States. Since obesity is a modifiable risk factor for coronary artery disease, we sought to determine whether body mass index (BMI) is an independent predictor of adverse in-hospital outcomes in patients with acute ST-elevation myocardial infarction (STEMI) treated with primary percutaneous coronary intervention (PPCI).

METHODS: We compared the outcome of all consecutive patients with STEMI, stratified by BMI (normal < 25 kg/m^2, $N = 36$; overweight 25 to 29.9 kg/m^2, $N = 62$; and obese ≥ 30 kg/m^2, $N = 41$) who underwent PPCI. Multivariable logistic regression analysis was performed to identify the independent predictive role of BMI for death.

RESULTS: There were 139 patients, aged 59 ± 13 years, treated with PPCI. Mean BMI for the obese group was 35 ± 6 kg/m^2 ($p < .001$ vs. each of the other two groups). Baseline clinical characteristics were similar among the three weight groups, except for a lower age and a higher rate of hyperlipidemia among the obese group ($p < .01$ for both). In-hospital death occurred in 17%, 10%, and 7%, respectively ($p = .20$). Renal failure occurred more often in the normal BMI group ($p = .02$). By multivariable analysis, BMI was not an independent predictor of in-hospital mortality. The only independent predictor of in-hospital mortality was diabetes mellitus ($p = .02$).

CONCLUSION: This study suggests that BMI is not an independent predictor of in-hospital mortality. These findings do not negate the need for sustained secondary prevention of obesity and its cardiac consequences.

courses beyond initial basic biostatistics. To further attain a strong foundation in statistics and to support faculty who may be less comfortable with statistics, RMU hired a part-time PhD-prepared statistical consultant who is available to students and faculty on an individual basis throughout the capstone process. In addition, the statistician offers workshops each semester open to both students and faculty. This model for maximizing statistical proficiency has strengthened capstone projects. Course objectives for the course *Statistics in Health Care* are in this basic course and threaded throughout the BSN-DNP curriculum (Figure 2.4).

An example of a capstone project that reflects the level of statistical analysis appropriate for a DNP capstone project is displayed in Figure 2.5.

CONCLUSION

While many DNP programs require publication-ready manuscripts as benchmarks for program outcomes, the focus of the DNP capstone is not congruent with many data-based, peer reviewed research journals. Rather, the capstone project is a process through which the BSN-DNP student gains a clear understanding of patient outcomes and the multiple factors that impact delivery of patient care. The capstone project should generate questions, stimulate critical evidence-based thinking, and encourage health policy development that enhances patient care and population health. This process gives the DNP nurse the opportunity to advance to a place of prominence within health care teams at the institutional and at the national level. With strong translational research skills, the DNP nurse is a leader who is empowered to move to the head of the table.

REFERENCES

American Academy of Nursing. (2010). *Implementing health care reform: Issues for nursing.* Retrieved from http://www.aannet.org/assets/docs/implementinghealthcarereform.pdf

American Association of Colleges of Nursing. (2004). *Position statement on the practice doctorate in nursing.* Retrieved from http://www.aacn.nche.edu/DNP/DNPPositionStatement.htm

American Association of Colleges of Nursing. (2006). *The essentials of doctoral education for advanced nursing practice.* Retrieved from http://www.aacn.nche.edu/publications/position/DNPEssentials.pdf

American Association of Colleges of Nursing. (2013). *DNP factsheet.* Retrieved from http://www.aacn.nche.edu/media-relations/fact-sheets/dnp

Institute of Medicine. (2010). *The future of nursing: Leading change, advancing health.* Washington, DC: National Academy of Sciences Press.

National Committee for Quality Assurance. (2005). *NCQA annual report 2005: Common ground, common goals.* Washington, DC: Author.

National Organization of Nurse Practitioner Faculties. (2012). *NP core competencies.* Retrieved from http://www.nonpf.org/?page=14

United States Department of Health and Human Services. (2010). *About the law.* Retrieved from http://www.hhs.gov/healthcare/rights/index.html

3

The DNP *Essentials* and the Evidence-Based Practice Framework: Foundations of a Capstone Exemplar

Pamela Lusk, Bernadette Mazurek Melnyk, and Lynn Gallagher Ford

The doctor of nursing practice (DNP) is a rigorous and demanding *practice-focused* doctoral program, designed to "prepare experts in advanced nursing practice" (American Association of Colleges of Nursing [AACN], 2006, p. 3). DNP education is heavily focused on innovative and evidence-based practices (EBPs) that reflect the ability to translate research findings to practice settings. Unlike the PhD-prepared nurse who generates external evidence through rigorous research, the DNP-prepared nurse generates internal evidence through quality improvement, outcomes management, and EBP change projects (Melnyk et al., 2013). Further, the DNP provides leadership in the advanced practice of nursing and demonstrates competence in knowledge activities, particularly "the translation of research into practice and the dissemination and evaluation of new knowledge" (AACN, 2006, p. 11). This reflects the core requirement that the DNP be highly knowledged in the EBP process as well as the ability to lead and support others in evidence-based care.

EBP AND THE DNP *ESSENTIALS*

The DNP *Essentials* (AACN, 2006) describe eight foundational competencies that are core to all advanced practice nursing roles. Several of the *Essentials* contain language that calls for DNP education to be structured with EBP as a central proficiency and expectation of the DNP graduate. The most pertinent ones are listed below.

DNP Essential I: Scientific Underpinnings for Practice

A wide array of scientific knowledge required by the DNP is addressed, and the DNP must not only possess such knowledge, but must also have the ability to translate knowledge quickly and efficiently to benefit patients in practice environments. Science is translated into practice through the EBP process.

DNP Essential II: Organizational and Systems Leadership for Quality Improvement and Systems Thinking

Proficiency in organizational and systems leadership is addressed. The DNP scope is distinguished by proficiency in conceptualizing new care models related to direct care, various populations, and communities of care. These conceptualizations of care are expected to be based in contemporary nursing science and evaluated in terms of feasibility within current organizational, political, cultural, and economic perspectives. Examination of new approaches to care and determining their feasibility in practice settings are both addressed through the EBP process. This *Essential* also requires that the DNP be proficient in creating and sustaining measurable changes within organizations in order to improve quality. DNPs are expected to make practice change recommendations, utilize principles of economics and finance to redesign care delivery systems, and proficiently evaluate the cost effectiveness of recommendations for change. All of these attributes are built into the EBP process, appraising current evidence to make practice change recommendations, feasibly integrating evidence into practice to improve the quality of care, evaluating outcomes of practice changes implemented, and disseminating findings from practice change projects and contributing to the body of knowledge to inform practice in the future.

DNP Essential III: Clinical Scholarship and Analytical Methods for EBP

EBP as a central role and skill of the DNP is directly addressed. In this *Essential*, key activities of the DNP are defined within scholarship and include application of knowledge to solve problems through the translation of research into practice and the dissemination and integration of new knowledge. Although the construct of EBP is reflected most directly in this *Essential*, it also is found in several other *Essentials*.

DNP Essential V: Health Care Policy for Advocacy in Health Care

The DNP role is described as including a broad advocacy role on behalf of the public through design, influence, and implementation of health care policies related to financing, practice regulation, safety, and quality. The DNP provides interface between practice, research, and policy. The EBP process includes consideration of these same key contributing factors: practice, research (evidence), and policy (patient or population impacted).

DNP Essential VII: Clinical Prevention and Population Health for Improving the Nation's Health

The DNP graduate is described as having a foundation in clinical prevention and population health. This foundation requires the ability to analyze scientific data, synthesize concepts, and develop/implement/evaluate interventions to address a continuum of care related to health promotion, disease prevention, and gaps in care. The EBP process is an ideal framework for the work required to meet this *Essential*.

DNP Essential VIII: Advanced Practice Nursing

The DNP graduate is required to practice (design, implement, and evaluate therapeutic interventions) in his or her advanced role based on the application of multiple sciences appropriate to their subspecialty. The DNP is expected to demonstrate advanced levels of critical judgment, systems thinking, and accountability in providing evidence-based care to improve patient outcomes. The EBP process is the foundation for advanced practice decision making and thoughtful selection of interventions to provide the best care to improve patient outcomes.

FRAMEWORK FOR THE DNP CAPSTONE

Doctoral education in nursing is intended to prepare nurses for the highest level of leadership in both practice and scientific inquiry. Whether enrolled in a research-focused doctoral program (PhD) or a practice-focused doctoral program (DNP), students are expected to demonstrate the following two attributes: ". . . a scholarly approach to the discipline and a commitment to the advancement of the profession" (AACN, 2006, p. 3). A critical differentiator between research-focused doctorate (PhD) graduates and the practice-focused doctorate (DNP) graduates is a clear sense of what these individuals *do in health care* once they have graduated. Therefore, it makes sense that the content included in these two types of doctoral programs as well as the final product generated by students in these programs would be very different from one another. There are distinctly unique mechanisms for the PhD student and the DNP student to demonstrate the attributes of doctorally prepared nurses. Research-focused programs generally require the student to carry out a rigorous, original extensive research study that is reported in a dissertation. On the other hand, practice-focused programs generally require the student to carry out a capstone project as the terminal work of the DNP.

Students entering DNP programs are introduced to *The Essentials of Doctoral Education for Advanced Nursing Practice* (AACN, 2006). The DNP clinical scholarly project should demonstrate the student's achievement of the eight *Essentials* (Moran, Conrad, & Burson, 2014). The capstone project is designed to reflect all of the *Essentials* in a single, grand project that is developed and built upon as the DNP student progresses through the advanced education program. The capstone project should serve as a synthesis of a student's work and a platform for future scholarship after graduation. There is a wide variety of DNP final products that can be produced; however, a single theme that is required of the DNP scholarly project is "the use of evidence to improve either practice or patient outcomes" (AACN, 2006, p. 20).

The DNP capstone project and the framework to support it should be intentionally designed to dovetail with the expected outcomes of the DNP program. The framework for designing exemplary capstone projects should include mechanisms for all of the *Essentials* to be demonstrated. However, frameworks can be invented when it makes sense to borrow from work that has already been established and tested. The seven steps of EBP form a simple step-by-step process that can serve well as a capstone framework. The overarching requirement of EBP proficiency for the DNP graduate is reinforced by the continuous utilization of the EBP process and the comprehensive application of the steps of the process, which affords opportunities for the integration and demonstration of all of the *Essentials*.

The seven steps of EBP provide a process whereby the advanced practice registered nurse (APRN) can find the best evidence to answer clinical practice questions, apply what has been learned to the clinical setting, and measure and evaluate the outcomes of a practice change based on the best evidence. Although challenges typically come with changing practice in health care systems, changes based on the best evidence result in the APRN providing improved care and gaining the confidence of knowing that one's patients are routinely receiving the best, most effective intervention available (Lusk & Melnyk, 2011a).

CAPSTONE EXEMPLAR: AN EBP CHANGE

This capstone exemplar was completed at a University College of Nursing where the curriculum is based on the EBP paradigm: changing one's practice from "usual care" (care that is steeped in tradition) to EBP that can improve patient outcomes and professional practice (Melnyk & Fineout-Overholt, 2011). As advanced practice psychiatric nurses (APPNs) routinely provide care to their clients, compelling questions arise about whether the treatments they are providing are the best practices. This exemplar describes how a DNP student was guided to design and implement an EBP capstone project from beginning clinical inquiry to dissemination of the results of the completed project.

This capstone, titled *The Brief Cognitive-Behavioral COPE Intervention for Depressed Adolescents: Outcomes and Feasibility of Delivery in 30-Minute Outpatient Visits*, was primarily built upon clinical scholarship (see *Essential III—Clinical Scholarship and Analytical Methods for Evidence-Based Practice.*) However, the other seven *Essentials* were addressed as well. The seven steps of EBP were used as the framework for this DNP project example (see Table 3.1).

TABLE 3.1 *The Seven Steps of Evidence-Based Practices (Melnyk & Fineout-Overholt, 2011)*

	Step
0	Cultivate a spirit of inquiry
1	Ask the burning question in PICOT format
2	Search for and collect the most relevant best evidence
3	Critically appraise the evidence
4	Integrate the best evidence with one's clinical expertise and patient preferences and values in making a practice decision or change
5	Evaluate outcomes of the practice decision or change based on evidence
6	Disseminate the outcomes of the evidence-based practice decision or change

Cultivate a Spirit of Inquiry

Engaging student interest in and excitement for the EBP process is critical. The role of the faculty mentor is central in capitalizing on students' natural spirit of inquiry regarding clinical practice issues and then guiding them in becoming proficient in the EBP process. A mentor can also facilitate growth throughout the DNP program, as DNP students achieve competency with the *Essentials* and progress from a primarily clinical practice role to the expanded DNP role.

The faculty mentor who directed this capstone project exemplar, Dr. Bernadette Melnyk, is an expert in EBP and also an expert in child/adolescent mental health, my area of clinical interest. From our initial meeting the focus was on the goal. Dr. Melnyk asked, "How do you want to make a big difference in outcomes for the adolescents and children who have mental health needs?" We began by discussing the prevalence of clinical depression in adolescents and our concern that so few adolescents who need treatment for depression receive any treatment at all (see *Essential VII—Clinical Prevention and Population Health for Improving the Nation's Health*). Teens are suffering with depressive symptoms that interfere with their optimal functioning at school, at home, and in social settings even though there are effective, evidence-based treatments for depression. Dr. Melnyk always addressed immediate questions, but then would remind me to think big, "What is your dream, your big vision for improving outcomes for these young people?" (see *Essential V—Health Care Policy for Advocacy in Health Care*). Acknowledged DNP expert, Lisa Chism, purports, "DNP graduates are positioned to be powerful advocates for health care policy through their practice experience" (Chism, 2012, p. 18).

This vision of providing adolescents with the best EBP for depression not only sustained my energy and passion for the DNP project but also informed the design of the project. We talked about the possibilities for a project that would answer not only the burning clinical questions I had, but would also be applicable to other clinical settings caring for depressed adolescents. We reviewed psychological theories of depression and psychotherapy supported by sound scientific studies (see *Essential I—Scientific Underpinnings for Practice*). We shared knowledge of current clinical guidelines for treatment of depressed adolescents and we discussed trends in the current practice of psychiatric mental health nurse practitioners (PMHNPs).

In our initial meeting Dr. Melnyk asked me directly, "What do you do in your practice? Do you provide the best evidence-based interventions?" The question was profound. I knew that I was not routinely providing the best evidence-based treatment in my practice with adolescents in a rural community mental health center. I was primarily conducting psychiatric evaluations and managing medications. This question ignited my determination to seek out current evidence supporting best treatment approaches for depressed teens and to develop a plan for initiating and evaluating EBP. As I explored reasons why I did not routinely provide psychotherapy sessions at my community mental health clinic (such as tightly scheduled 30-minute medication management visits), I became aware of the need to involve other members of the treatment and administrative team in addressing change at the organizational level (see *Essential II—Organizational and Systems Leadership for Quality Improvement and Systems Thinking*).

As we established a mentor–student working relationship, Dr. Melnyk and I clarified expectations. We agreed to meet regularly, approximately every 6 weeks, face to face. I would be responsible for letting Dr. Melnyk know when DNP course assignments would need her input (such as the institutional review process [IRB] application). I learned to bring a clear agenda to our meetings so that our time was used efficiently. Some of the most perceptive questions she asked during the development of the capstone project were:

- "Why is there a gap in what we know, and what is usual care?"
- "What do you see as barriers for providing the best evidence-based care in your *real-world* population?"
- "Are these common barriers that other APPNs and clinicians face?"
- "What are your ideas for addressing those barriers and changing practice to provide evidence-based interventions for all the adolescents who badly need help?"

I left our meetings thinking more broadly, considering new ideas, and with strengthened resolve to move forward in the EBP process with my capstone. "The mentor's exquisite listening" can lead to identifying obstacles you could not see (Heinrich, 2008, p. 166). Gaps in the plan can be pointed out and strategies formed to address barriers. The mentor can share examples of how to address challenges when designing and implementing EBP projects. The mentor can also discern if the student has an ability to maintain an objective view of the topic.

With skilled inquiry by the mentor, we refined the "burning question" to be addressed in the project. Through this process we designed an appropriate and meaningful clinical scholarly project, i.e., the DNP capstone. The mentor always kept the vision in the forefront, stating: "Your DNP project can help many young people get the treatment they need. We will improve the mental health treatment for adolescents" (see *Essential V—Health Care Policy for Advocacy in Health Care*). A positive synergistic working relationship with a respected faculty mentor inspires and energizes the student to develop a project that has the potential to make a difference.

Ask the Burning Clinical Question in PICOT Format

Each component of the PICOT question must be thoughtfully considered to formulate a well-articulated question, critical to searching for the best evidence (Melnyk & Fineout-Overholt, 2011). My clinical inquiry was then transformed into a searchable, answerable question using PICOT format:

- P – patient population
- I – intervention or issue of interest
- C – comparison intervention
- O – outcome to be measured
- T – time frame

The mentor's role in this step is essential. Chism (2012) describes the role of the capstone mentor in formulating the question:

> A mentor's assessment of the student's knowledge, experience and abilities can lead to a project that will fit within the time frame of the program and meet the criteria for a quality doctoral clinical scholarly project. DNP project mentors clarify the questions being raised, set boundaries on the scope of the project and ensure that the data [that] will be collected will yield valid and reliable information pertinent to the question being asked as well as making sure ethical standards are met. (p. 114)

My PICOT question for this project to guide the search for evidence was:

- In depressed adolescents (P) . . .
- how does cognitive-behavioral therapy (CBT; I) . . .
- versus usual care (C) . . .
- improve depressive symptoms (O) . . .
- over a 3-month period (T)?

Search For and Collect the Most Relevant, Best Evidence

Based on the initial search utilizing the PICOT question, additional keywords were identified to enhance the breadth and depth of the search. Because the PICOT question for this project was an intervention question, the *Cochrane Database of Systematic Reviews* was an appropriate place to begin the search. This strategy resulted in a systematic review of randomized controlled trials (RCTs) by Watanabe, Hunot, Omori, Churchill, and Farukawa (2007) that reviewed studies of psychotherapy effectiveness for children and adolescents with depression. In the next step in the search, MEDLINE, PsycINFO, and CINAHL were searched. Several meta-analyses were located on the topic of treatment of adolescent depression. Literature review saturation point was reached when the same studies kept coming up in the various meta-analyses. The search continued with *National Guideline Clearinghouse* for practice guidelines to treat depression in adolescents.

Critically Appraise the Evidence (Rapid Critical Appraisal, Evaluation, and Synthesis)

The systematic review by Watanabe and colleagues (2007) supported CBT and interpersonal psychotherapy as effective treatments for adolescents with depression. In the search of PsycINFO and other databases, several meta-analyses of RCTs, including McCarty and Weisz (2007), supported CBT as an effective treatment for depressed adolescents. McCarty and Weisz (2007) identified the components of CBT that are present in effective CBT interventions with depressed adolescents. One of the RCTs, *The Treatment of Adolescent Depression Study (TADS)* by March et al. (2007), was a landmark 13-site RCT that compared CBT, placebo, antidepressant medication (fluoxetine), and a combination of fluoxetine and CBT. The study determined the superior effectiveness of the combination of CBT and fluoxetine in both acute and continuation treatment of adolescent major depression.

Critical appraisal of each of the studies included an assessment of their validity and applicability to practice as described by Melnyk and Fineout-Overholt (2011). After a critical appraisal of each study, the findings were synthesized in order to assess the strength of the body of evidence to make a practice change.

The literature review indicated that some of the studies provided strong Level 1 evidence (the strongest level of evidence to guide practice, and included a systematic review and a meta-analysis of RCTs) and Level 2 evidence from the TADS RCT (the strongest study design for controlling extraneous or confounding variables) to support CBT as a very efficacious treatment for adolescent depression. In reviewing the studies included in meta-analysis, when specified, individual CBT sessions were 60 minutes in length. Group CBT programs for adolescents were also included in the meta-analysis. Cited CBT treatment manuals for depressed adolescents were obtained and reviewed for applicability to brief sessions. In the treatment manuals reviewed, all authors recommended the individual sessions be 60 minutes. The evidence review provided clear direction for the best evidence-based treatment for adolescent depression.

Earlier in her academic career, my mentor had developed a cognitive-behavioral skills building program, *Creating Opportunities for Personal Empowerment* (COPE), that had been piloted with overweight teens in group and school settings (Melnyk et al., 2007, 2009). The COPE program included all of the components of effective CBT programs for depressed adolescents, as identified in a meta-analysis by McCarty and Weisz (2007).

COPE trainings have been offered at the College of Nursing and at national conferences for clinicians/teachers working with adolescents and families. The COPE program is currently being delivered in many middle and high schools throughout the nation, in pediatric practices, primary care practices, as well as in outpatient and inpatient psychiatric specialty services. A recent full-scale RCT was conducted with 779 high school teens, incorporating the COPE cognitive-behavioral skills-building program into a 15-session comprehensive healthy lifestyle intervention (i.e., the COPE Healthy Lifestyles TEEN [Thinking, Emotions, Exercise, and Nutrition] Program) into the required health course (Melnyk et al., 2013).

Findings from this study indicated that students who received the COPE Healthy Lifestyles TEEN program, in comparison to those who received an attention control program, had higher levels of physical activity, less progression from normal weight to overweight, better social skills, and higher academic performance. In addition, COPE students who started the program with severe depression had normal levels of depressive symptoms after the program in comparison to attention-control students whose depressive symptoms remained elevated (Melnyk et al., 2013).

Integrate the Best Evidence With Clinical Expertise and Patient Preferences and Values in Making a Practice Decision or Change

The COPE program was selected as the EBP change for this project. A crucial aspect of project design was to ensure that the COPE intervention could be delivered within the time constraints of the 30-minute outpatient medication management. Many NPs are practicing in community mental health centers with 15- to 30-minute medication checks as the norm (Wheeler, 2014, p. xxvi). Because of the shortage of child and adolescent psychiatric providers, efficient use of clinician time is a priority. As the content of these sessions is concise and fits well within the 30-minute appointment time, I proposed that this time frame was sufficient for psychotherapy, ongoing assessment, and medication management.

It is poor practice to maintain long waitlists for psychiatric evaluation. At agencies with insufficient child psychiatric providers, there is now an emphasis on brief, focused (short-term) interventions, allowing many adolescents who need treatment to get started and receive treatment in a timely fashion. The COPE sessions are designed to be presented in a seven-session Teen Manual (see *Essential III—Clinical Scholarship and Analytical Methods for Evidence-Based Practice*). The limit of seven sessions allows teens to move in and out of intervention quickly, so more teens can also have access to active, evidence-based treatment.

Through prior education I had knowledge and skills to conduct cognitive behavioral therapy, and Dr. Melnyk trained me to deliver the COPE program. Each COPE session was audio taped, with teen assent and parental consent. I presented some trial COPE sessions to teens already in treatment (with permission from parent and teen) and the response was very positive. The teens liked the focus on lessons with teen examples and their parents found the materials appropriate for the teen's developmental level. Both the teens and parents indicated that the COPE content spoke to concerns adolescents commonly express about their functioning at home, at school, and in social situations. The teens also responded well to the skills-building activities and indicated that they were helpful. In outpatient mental health practice, it is common for parents to bring their child or adolescent for evaluation and treatment, stating they do not want their young person started on antidepressant medication. When parents expressed this clear preference and shared their values about what is acceptable treatment, these preferences were incorporated into the plan of care.

With guidance from my mentor, I anticipated questions and concerns that the leadership team at my site might have. I negotiated with both clinical and organizational leadership to implement the seven sessions of the COPE program within the usual 30-minute visit, with additional follow-up for each teen in the project (see *Essential II—Organizational and Systems Leadership for Quality Improvement and Systems Thinking*). The rationale was the strong evidence supporting the combination of psychotherapy in addition to medication management as the best practices approach for treating adolescent depression.

I gave information to the medical director about both the COPE materials and evidence supporting utilization of a CBT-based program. We discussed how the process would work with each teen, including the informed consent process. The medical director was pleased that COPE was limited to seven sessions and one post-COPE evaluation session, enabling more teens to be reached. The medical director then invited me to explain the COPE materials at a medical staff meeting. The psychiatry team asked why we were not offering this intervention to all of the teens (see *Essential VI—Interprofessional Collaboration for Improving Patient and Population Health Outcomes*).

In response to my presentation, the chief clinical administrator stated, "You know I have always valued psychotherapy, but we have no way to pay for it." Fortunately, my mentor and I had anticipated that cost would be an important consideration for clinic administration and had prepared a cost analysis. In discussion with billers and coders at the clinic business office, I determined that the COPE sessions could be coded and billed as *Psychotherapy/Counseling and Evaluation and Management*, delivered within the usual 30-minute medication-management appointment by a "medical" provider. By using this code for psychotherapy/counseling in face-to-face encounters for more than 50% of visits, the PMHNP would be billing at a higher rate. The billers agreed to track COPE session bills to determine whether or not third-party payers reimbursed for the services.

Using the clinic computerized scheduling and billing system involved meeting with stakeholders in the front office staff and in the management-coding-billing department to ensure that the current electronic health record was compatible with the proposed visit format (see *Essential II—Organizational and Systems Leadership for Quality Improvement and Systems Thinking* and *Essential IV—Information Systems/Technology and Patient Care Technology for the Improvement and Transformation of Health Care*). The plan to address agency cost concerns was very instrumental in getting full leadership team approval and the letter of support needed for submission to the University IRB.

Leadership also agreed on a follow-up plan for the COPE teens. They would be followed by the PMHNP after the intervention concluded, on an ongoing, as-needed basis. The COPE Teen DNP project was deemed consistent with the agency's mission of providing excellence in psychiatric care (see *Essential II—Organizational and Systems Leadership for Quality Improvement and Systems Thinking*).

Evaluate Outcomes of the Practice Decision or Change Based on Evidence

To determine whether COPE would be effective for the depressed teens seen in this clinical setting, an outcome evaluation was planned. The outcome measure, using the *Beck Youth Depression Inventory*, was improvement in depressive symptoms. The others are also included. The teens easily fill out these inventories in about 5 minutes each. There were 25 self-reported items to circle using a Likert scale of *never, sometimes, often*, or *always* for each item. The Beck Inventories have reliability and excellent internal consistency reliability, and are normed for girls and boys ages 7 to 18 years (Beck, Beck, Jolly, & Steer, 2005).

A *Personal Beliefs* scale, developed by Dr. Melnyk, was administered pre- and postintervention, and both parents and teens were asked to fill out post-COPE evaluation forms. These evaluation forms were open-ended, with questions such as: *What did you find most helpful in the COPE program?* Responses were anonymous. The intent of the open-ended questionnaires was to gain information about ways to improve delivery of COPE, and to determine if this intervention was acceptable to the wide age range of teens (from 12-year-old middle school students to seniors in high school). It also allowed the teens and parents the opportunity to provide feedback about the COPE experience.

The COPE program was delivered by an APPN in individual 30-minute sessions at the community mental health clinic. Fifteen teens met criteria for depression and enrolled in the COPE project (during the length of the study), completing all seven sessions. Adolescents reported significant decreases in depression, anxiety, anger, and destructive behavior as well as increases in self-concept and personal beliefs about managing negative emotions (Lusk & Melnyk, 2011b). Evaluations indicated that COPE was a positive experience for teens and parents. Third-party payers reimbursed for the COPE sessions.

Disseminate the Outcome of the EBP Decision or Change

This project was disseminated at national conferences and in publications in peer-reviewed journals. My mentor shared her experiences with presenting and publishing, providing excellent role modeling at conference presentations. The presentations have been enthusiastically received. Disseminating the findings from the capstone project through national presentations and publications has resulted in rapid translation of the evidence-based COPE intervention into practice settings, aiming to improve outcomes for high-risk adolescents.

IMPACT

This DNP capstone project used the seven steps of EBP and selected *Essentials* to implement an EBP change, resulting in improved outcomes for depressed teens treated at a rural community-based mental health clinic. In addition, I routinely offer COPE to all adolescents who present with depression and/or anxiety at the primary care clinic where I practice. This is an integration of mental health care with primary care, working collaboratively with the pediatric clinicians. As a focused, brief intervention, clinics using COPE can increase access to evidence-based treatment for teens and families. Clinicians can be trained to deliver the seven sessions promoting program sustainability. Lastly, it is a cost-effective intervention and third-party payers have demonstrated willingness to pay for this service. This capstone impacts population health and promotes the nation's health (see *Essential VII—Population Health for Improving the Nation's Health*).

REFERENCES

American Association of Colleges of Nursing. (2006). *The essentials of doctoral education for advanced nursing practice*. Retrieved from http://www.aacn.nche.edu/publications/position/DNPEssentials.pdf

Beck, J. S., Beck, A. T., Jolly, J. B., & Steer, R. A. (2005). *Beck Youth Inventories second edition manual (BYI-II)*. San Antonio, TX: Pearson.

Chism, L. A. (2012). *The doctor of nursing practice: A guidebook for role development and professional issues* (2nd ed.). Burlington, MA: Jones & Bartlett Learning.

Heinrich, K. T. (2008). *A nurse's guide to presenting and publishing: Dare to share.* Sudbury, MA: Jones & Bartlett.

Lusk, P., & Melnyk, B. M. (2011a). COPE for the treatment of depressed adolescents: Lessons learned from implementing an evidence-based practice change. *Journal of the American Psychiatric Nurses Association, 17*(4), 297–309. doi:10.1177/1078390311416117

Lusk, P., & Melnyk, B. M. (2011b). The brief cognitive-behavioral COPE intervention for depressed adolescents: Outcomes and feasibility of delivery in 30-minute outpatient visits. *Journal of the American Psychiatric Nurses Association, 17*(3), 226–236. doi:10.1177/1078390311404067

March, J. S., Silva, S., Petrycki, S., Curry, J., Wells, K., Fairbank, J., . . . Severe, J. (2007). The Treatment of Adolescents With Depression Study (TADS): Long term effectiveness and safety outcomes. *Archives of General Psychiatry, 64*(10), 1132–1143. doi:10.1001/archpsyc.64.10.1132

McCarty, C. A., & Weisz, J. R. (2007). Effects of psychotherapy for depression in children and adolescents: What we can (and can't) learn from meta-analysis and component profiling. *Journal of the American Academy of Child and Adolescent Psychiatry, 46*(7), 879–886. doi:10.1097/chi.0b013e31805467b3

Melnyk, B., & Fineout-Overholt, E. (2011). *Evidence-based practice in nursing & healthcare: A guide to best practice* (2nd ed.). Baltimore, MD: Wolters Kluwer.

Melnyk, B. M., Jacobson, D., Kelly, S., Belyea, M., Shaibi, G., Small, L., . . . Marsiglia, F. F. (2013). Promoting healthy lifestyles in high school adolescents: A randomized controlled trial. *American Journal of Preventive Medicine, 45*(4), 407–415. doi:10.1016/j.amepre.2013.05.013

Melnyk, B. M., Jacobson, D., Kelly, S., O'Haver, J., Small, L., & Mays, M. Z. (2009). Improving the mental health, healthy lifestyle choices, and physical health of Hispanic adolescents: A randomized controlled pilot study. *Journal of School Health, 79*(12), 575–584. doi:10.1111/j.1746-1561.2009.00451.x

Melnyk, B. M., Small, L., Morrison-Beedy, D., Strasser, A., Spath, L., Kreipe, R., . . . O'Haver, J. (2007). The COPE healthy lifestyles TEEN program: Feasibility, preliminary efficacy, & lessons learned from an after school group intervention with overweight adolescents. *Journal of Pediatric Health Care, 21*(5), 315–322. doi:10.1016/j.pedhc.2007.02.009

Moran, K. J., Conrad, D., & Burson, R. (2014). *The doctor of nursing practice scholarly project: A framework for success.* Burlington, MA: Jones & Bartlett.

Watanabe, N., Hunot, V., Omori, I. M., Churchill, R., & Farukawa, T. A. (2007). Psychotherapy for depression among children and adolescents: A systematic review. *Acta Psychiatrica Scandinavica, 116*(2), 84–95. doi:10.1111/j.1600-0447.2007.01018.x

Wheeler, K. (2014). *Psychotherapy for the advanced practice psychiatric nurse: A how-to guide for evidence-based practice* (2nd ed.). New York, NY: Springer Publishing Company.

DNP Exemplars: Excellence in Practice

Excellence is never an accident. It is always the result of high intention, sincere effort, and intelligent execution.

—Aristotle

4

Burnout as a Barrier to Practice Among Nurse–Midwives: Examining the Evidence

Rebeca Barroso

DNP Essential #1

Scientific underpinnings for practice

American Association of Colleges of Nursing. (2006). *The essentials of doctoral education for advanced nursing practice.* Retrieved from http://www.aacn.nche .edu/publications/position/DNPEssentials.pdf

The chapter describes burnout as a barrier to practice among nurse–midwives.
    It exemplifies DNP *Essential #1* as it relates to the application of evidence, the scientific underpinnings for practice, as the basis for explaining a clinical problem.

Barbara A. Anderson, Editor

CAPSTONE FOCUS

Burnout affects professionals in all clinical specialties (Maslach & Leiter, 2005), including nurse–midwives in clinical practice (Beaver, Sharp, & Cotsonis, 1986). This capstone project used scientific evidence to examine burnout among nurse–midwives. It also replicated the only published nurse–midwifery burnout study (Beaver et al., 1986).

REVIEW OF THE LITERATURE

The Prevalence of Burnout

The initial discussion of burnout, as a state of physical and emotional exhaustion secondary to workplace stressors, is credited to Freudenberger (1974). Burnout, as an occupational and workplace-generated phenomenon, has been extensively studied in the intervening years (Schaufeli, Leiter, & Maslach, 2009). Since the 1990s, occupational and workplace burnout has been considered a worldwide "pandemic" (Golembiewski, Boudreau, Munzenrider, & Luo, 1996). There are no consistent employment factors that contribute to burnout. Rather, burnout is related to organizational risk factors: workload, control, reward, community, values, and fairness (Maslach & Leiter, 2008).

The health and human services professions, and more specifically clinical practitioners, are at greatest risk for burnout (Afzal et al., 2010; Ballenger-Browning et al., 2011; Becker, Milad, & Klock, 2006; Buunk & Schaufeli, 1993; Burke & Greenglass, 2001; Dyrbye et al., 2010; Rosenberg & Pace, 2006; Schaufeli & Bakker, 2004; Vahey, Aiken, Sloan, Clarke, & Vargas, 2004). In the original nurse–midwife burnout study, more than 40% of the nurse–midwives reported moderate to high levels of burnout in the emotional exhaustion dimension (Beaver et al., 1986).

Burnout Defined

Burnout is a syndrome manifested by emotional exhaustion, depersonalization, and a reduced sense of personal accomplishment (Maslach & Jackson, 1981, 1986; Maslach, Jackson, & Leiter, 1997). Most recently, Maslach and Leiter (2008) defined burnout as "a continuum between the negative experience of burnout and the positive experience of engagement. . . with three interrelated dimensions. . . exhaustion-energy, cynicism-involvement, and inefficacy-efficacy" (p. 498). The basic individual emotional strain of burnout is the exhaustion component, which includes feeling overextended and depleted of both emotional and physical resources, and constitutes the most salient aspect of the syndrome. The authors describe the cynicism component as a negative, detached, uncaring response in the interpersonal context of the work. Inefficacy is manifested as feelings of lack of productivity, achievement, and incompetence. The inefficacy component is the most difficult to evaluate of the three burnout components (Maslach & Leiter, 2008).

Barriers Contributing to Burnout

Personal barriers associated with burnout among nurse–midwives in the original study included young age of the professional and child care responsibilities. Employment barriers included new employment in practice, low salaries, and a high number of births among socioeconomically disadvantaged patients in the clinical service (Beaver et al., 1986), as well as a hostile practice climate (Browning, Ryan, Thomas, Greenberg, & Rolniak, 2007; Gustaffson, Eriksson, Strandberg, & Norberg, 2010). These findings parallel studies in other health service professions (Afzal et al., 2010; Becker et al., 2006; Burke & Greenglass, 2001; Ernst, Messmer, Franco, & Gonzalez, 2004; Maslach et al., 1997; Rosenberg & Pace, 2006; Schaufeli & Bakker, 2004; Schaufeli & Buunk, 2003; Turnipseed, 1998; Vahey et al., 2004).

THE CAPSTONE PROJECT

This capstone replicated the 1986 national nurse–midwife study (Beaver et al., 1986). It re-examined the prevalence and magnitude of burnout among members of the American College of Nurse–Midwives (ACNM) currently in clinical practice in the state of Pennsylvania. Personal and employment factors associated with burnout were evaluated. This capstone project compared findings with the original study.

Study Design

This project used descriptive and cross-sectional design. Institutional Review Board approval was obtained from Frontier Nursing University (FNU) and the Division of Research of ACNM. In the original study of burnout among nurse–midwives, Maslach and Jackson (1981a) used the first edition of the Maslach Burnout Inventory (MBI), a tool designed to measure burnout in the human services professions. This tool is the most widely used instrument to measure burnout (Worley, Vassar, Wheeler, & Barnes, 2008). In the replication study, the third edition of the MBI was used, including the survey designed to specifically measure burnout in the human services professions (Maslach et al., 1997). Additional demographic and clinical practice questions similar to those included in the original study were included to evaluate whether or not previously noted barriers had changed over time. All ACNM member nurse–midwives active in Pennsylvania, as described below, were surveyed.

The Project Site and Sample

This project was conducted among Pennsylvania nurse–midwives in contrast to the inclusion in the original study of all ACNM member nurse–midwives in the United States. In comparison to clinical practice realities that exist elsewhere in the country, Pennsylvania nurse–midwives enjoy favorable working conditions (ACNM, 2008; Declerq, 2009; Goodman, 2007). Pennsylvania nurse–midwives receive reimbursement at 100% of the Medicaid Physician Fee Schedule, and private insurance payment is mandated. Direct access to nurse–midwifery care is required by law (ACNM, 2008). There are over 100 nurse–midwifery clinical practices in the state, ranging from solo practices to large hospital-based practices (ACNM, 2008).

State regulations and the political climate in Pennsylvania do not restrict nurse–midwifery clinical practice by birth setting (ACNM, 2008). There are nurse–midwives in Pennsylvania attending births at home, in free-standing birth centers, and in small and large hospitals (ACNM, 2011). In 2008, Pennsylvania midwives attended 12,075 vaginal births, representing 11.9% of the vaginal births in Pennsylvania during that year (Pennsylvania Department of Health, 2011). The Pennsylvania rate of midwife-attended births compares favorably with the national rate of 7.3% of all vaginal births in the United States attended by nurse–midwives in 2007 (Declerq, 2011).

Replication Project Outcome

At the time of this capstone project implementation, 336 nurse–midwives held current licensure in the state (Pennsylvania Board of Medicine, 2011) and 223 were active members in the ACNM (G. Hamilton, personal communication, January 26, 2011). Of 223 questionnaires sent by surface mail to active Pennsylvania ACNM members, 174 were returned (78.0%). Twenty-five respondents were excluded from the evaluated data due to not being in clinical practice, two were excluded due to incomplete data, and two declined inclusion. See Table 4.1 for demographic comparison of respondents in the original and the replicated study.

The vast majority of the respondents in the original study were under the age of 50 ($n = 89, 92.7\%$), in contrast to the replicated study's abundance of nurse–midwives over the age of 50 ($n = 77, 54.2\%$); and there were slightly more single ($n = 50, 51\%$) than married or partnered nurse–midwives ($n = 48, 49\%$) in the original study, in comparison to 79.7% ($n = 114$) of the replicated study sample being comprised of married or partnered nurse–midwives.

TABLE 4.1 *Demographic Comparison of Respondents in Original and Replicated Groups*

Personal and Employment Variables	Original Group 1982, *N* = 98	Replicated Group 2011, *N* = 145
Age ≤ 50 years	89 (92.7)	65 (45.8)
Married/partnered	48 (49.0)	114 (79.7)
Child-care arrangements		
Somewhat of a problem	27 (55.1)	27 (35.1)
Frequently or always a problem	6 (12.2)	18 (23.4)
Education level		
Master's or doctorally prepared	47 (48.0)	128 (88.3)
Certificate, no graduate degree	51 (52.0)	17 (11.7)
Urban setting	75 (77.3)	66 (45.5)
Employment		
Public sector	35 (37.3)	48 (33.3)
Private practice	32 (34.0)	101 (70.1)
Nurse–midwife–owned practice	20 (20.4)	15 (10.4)
Out-of-hospital practice	16 (16.8)	34 (24.3)

A striking difference between the two studies is noted in terms of highest education. Whereas in the original study 48% ($n = 47$) of the nurse–midwives had earned a master's degree and none held a doctorate degree, in the replicated study, 88.2% ($n = 128$) of the nurse–midwives had earned a master's degree or higher.

The most salient unchanged personal demographic among the nurse–midwives in the original study and the replicated study is child-care arrangement. For those nurse–midwives with children at home, problems with child care persisted in the replicated study ($n = 45$, 31%), nearly equal in measure to the original study ($n = 33$, 34%).

In the original study, the nurse–midwives were working predominantly in urban settings ($n = 75$, 77.3%) while the nurse–midwives in the replicated study were working in near equal measures in urban ($n = 66$, 45.5%), suburban ($n= 78$, 53.8%), and rural settings ($n = 67$, 46.2%).

In comparing the types of institutions where the nurse–midwives work, there are similarities and differences in these two studies. In the original study group, 37.3% ($n = 35$) of the nurse–midwives were working in the public sector. Similarly, nearly 30 years later, 33.3% ($n = 48$) of the replicated study's nurse–midwives were working in the public sector. In contrast, in the original study only 34% ($n = 32$) of the nurse–midwives were working in private practices, while 70.1% ($n = 101$) of the nurse–midwives in the replicated study were working in private practices.

In 1982, 20.4% ($n = 20$) of the nurse–midwife respondents in the original study stated working in nurse–midwife–owned practices, while in 2011 the numbers of nurse–midwives in the replicated study that were working in such practices had nearly halved, to slightly over 10% (10.4%, $n = 15$). By contrast, there had been growth in out-of-hospital births: out-of-hospital births were being attended by 24.3% ($n =34$) of the replicated study nurse–midwives, in comparison to 16.8% ($n = 16$) in the original study group.

Burnout stress is closely associated with the level of perceived social support. See Table 4.2 for comparison of sources of stress and support among the original and replicated samples.

The nurse–midwives in the original study listed consumers/clients ($n = 92$, 93.9%), parents ($n = 78$, 79.6%), and nurses ($n = 74$, 75.5%) as their three top sources of support. Consumers/clients were also listed by the replicated study, but friends ($n = 125$, 87.4%) and colleague nurse–midwives ($n = 124$, 86.7%) were the two most frequently cited sources of support. Nurses, however, occupied third place as sources of support for the nurse–midwives in both the original ($n = 74$, 75.5%) and the replicated ($n = 120$, 83.9%) studies.

In the national study, nurse–midwives cited legislative concerns ($n = 49$, 50%), prescriptive privileges ($n = 33$, 33.7%), and hospital privileges ($n = 31$, 31.6%) as sources of stress with reimbursement ($n = 56$, 57.1%) as the main source of stress. Of these four most frequently cited sources of stress, the only one that was shared by the replicated study of nurse–midwives was the concern for the reimbursement cycle ($n = 43$, 30.1%), which was identified as a less frequent stressor than administrators ($n = 72$, 50.3%), physicians ($n = 69$, 48.3%), and nurses ($n = 44$, 30.8%).

TABLE 4.2 *Comparison of Support and Stress Sources*

Original Group, 1982 (*N* = 98)		Replicated Group, 2011 (*N* = 145)	
Sources of Support, *n* (%)		**Sources of Support, *n* (%)**	
Consumers/clients	92 (93.9)	Friends	125 (87.4)
Parent(s)	78 (79.6)	Nurse–midwives	124 (86.7)
Nurse(s)	74 (75.5)	Nurse(s)	120 (83.9)
Physicians	66 (67.3)	Spouse/partner	114 (79.7)
Community	64 (65.3)	Physicians	100 (69.9)
Spouse/partner	58 (59.2)	Consumers/clients	98 (68.5)
Sources of Stress, *n* (%)		**Sources of Stress, *n* (%)**	
Reimbursement cycle	56 (57.1)	Administrators	72 (50.3)
Legislative concerns	49 (50.0)	Physician(s)	69 (48.3)
Prescriptive concerns	33 (33.7)	Nurse(s)	44 (30.8)
Hospital privileges	31 (31.6)	Reimbursement cycle	43 (30.1)

Burnout Comparison

There were no statistically significant differences in the depersonalization and reduced personal accomplishment subscales between the nurse–midwives in the original study and the replicated study. There was a statistically significant difference between groups ($p = .02$) in the emotional exhaustion subscale, indicating that a statistically significant greater proportion of the replicated study nurse–midwives reported higher emotional exhaustion levels than was reported by the nurse–midwives in the original study.

Child-care arrangement difficulties remain a statistically significant intervening variable contributing to burnout among nurse–midwives. Four of the sources of support determined by Beaver et al. (1986) as contributing to reducing burnout in the original nurse–midwife sample were validated as statistically significant by the replicated nurse–midwife pilot study. Consistent with the original study's findings (Beaver et al., 1986), the replicated study nurse–midwives who received support from spouses/partners, clients, physicians, and legislators exhibited less burnout as evaluated in one or more of the MBI health services professions dimensions.

The replicated study yielded positive correlations between nurse–midwife burnout and worked intrapartum hours, on-call hours, and newborn/infant care hours. It also revealed an the association between burnout and full-time employment as a clinical nurse–midwife consistent with the Beaver et al. (1986) findings "as hours worked increased, burnout as measured by emotional exhaustion increased" (p. 8).

Other variables associated with increased burnout in the original nurse–midwife study were not confirmed by the replicated study. No associations were found in the replicated study between burnout and age, caring for young children at home, parental support, a high proportion of uninsured or underinsured clients, number of births, length of employment, and salaries as reported by Beaver et al. (1986).

IMPACT

The ACNM (2009) holds as one of its strategic priorities having nurse–midwives attending 20% of the vaginal births by the year 2020. In order to accomplish this goal, 1,000 new nurse–midwives must join the workforce every year by 2015, and great strides must be made to keep the current workforce in clinical practice longer (ACNM, 2009). The nurse–midwifery profession is rapidly aging, with over 24% of the current ACNM membership over the age of 64 (E. Moore, personal communication, December 27, 2013). The profession cannot afford to reduce the number or effectiveness of its members through the detrimental effects of burnout: compassion fatigue; job fatigue; and job dissatisfaction leading to disengagement, absenteeism, workplace instability, and attrition from the profession (Afzal et al., 2010; Ballenger et al., 2011; Becker et al., 2006; Browning et al., 2007; Dyrbye et al., 2010; Gustaffson et al., 2010; Rosenberg & Pace, 2006; Schaufeli et al., 2009; Vahey et al., 2004).

Nurse–midwives in clinical practice are adversely affected by burnout in the emotional dimension. The problem has remained largely unchanged over the last three decades, and the degree of emotional burnout could be advancing. The variables that have been identified as associated with nurse–midwife burnout provide more questions than answers. A literature search and focus groups are needed to begin to answer these questions. Using the findings gleaned from the replicated study and the findings of focus groups, a national study needs to be designed, funded, and implemented at the earliest possible time. At stake are the profession's goals for advancing the work of serving the health care needs of women, infants, and families.

REFERENCES

Afzal, K. I., Khan, F. M., Mulla, A., Akins, R., Leger, E., & Giordano, F. L. (2010). Primary language and cultural backgrounds as factors in resident burnout in medical specialties: A study in a bilingual US city. *Southern Medical Journal, 103*(7), 607–615. doi:10.1097/SMJ.0b013e3181e20cad

American College of Nurse–Midwives. (2008). *State fact sheets.* Retrieved from http://www.midwife.org/index.asp?bid=59&cat=11&button=Search&rec=211

American College of Nurse–Midwives. (2009). *ACNM future focus: Moving forward strategically to meet our long-term goals.* Retrieved from http://www.midwife.org/ACNM-Future-Focus

American College of Nurse–Midwives. (2011). *Online member and practice directory, Pennsylvania.* Retrieved from http://www.midwife.org/rp/online_practice.cfm

Ballenger-Browning, K. K., Schmitz, K. J., Rothacker, J. A., Hammer, P. S., Webb-Murphy, J. A., & Johnson, D. C. (2011). Predictors of burnout among military mental health providers. *Military Medicine, 176*(3), 253–260.

Beaver, R. C., Sharp, E. S., & Cotsonis, G. A. (1986). Burnout experienced by nurse–midwives. *Journal of Nurse–Midwifery, 31*(1), 3–15.

Becker, J. L., Milad, M. P., & Klock, S. C. (2006). Burnout, depression, and career satisfaction: Cross-sectional study of obstetrics and gynecology residents. *American Journal of Obstetrics and Gynecology, 195*(5), 1444–1449. doi:10.1016/j.ajog.2006.06.075

Browning, L., Ryan, C. S., Thomas, S., Greenberg, M., & Rolniak, S. (2007). Nursing specialty and burnout. *Psychology, Health & Medicine, 12*(2), 248–254. doi:10.1080/13548500600568290

Buunk, B. P., & Schaufeli, W. B. (1993). Professional burnout: A perspective from social comparison theory. In W. B. Schaufeli, C. Maaslach, & Y. T. Marek (Eds.), *Professional burnout: Recent developments in theory and research* (pp. 53–69). Washington, DC: Taylor & Francis.

Burke, R. J., & Greenglass, E. R. (2001). Hospital restructuring, work-family conflict and psychological burnout among nursing staff. *Psychology & Health, 16*(5), 583–594. doi:10.1080/08870440108405528

Declerq, E. (2009). Births attended by certified nurse–midwives in the United States reach an all-time high: Trends from 1986 to 2006. *Journal of Midwifery and Women's Health, 54*(3), 263–265. doi:10.1016/j.jmwh.2009.02.006

Declerq, E. (2011). Trend in midwife-attended births, 1989 to 2007. *Journal of Midwifery and Women's Health, 56*(2), 173–176. doi:10.1111/j.1542-2011.2011.00055.x

Dyrbye, L. N., Massie, F. S., Eacker, A., Harper, W., Power, D., Durning, S. J., . . .Shanafelt, T. D. (2010). Relationship between burnout and professional conduct and attitudes among US medical students. *The Journal of the American Medical Association, 304*(11), 1173–1180. doi:10.1001/jama.2010.1318

Ernst, M. E., Messmer, P. R., Franco, M., & Gonzalez, J. L. (2004). Nurses' job satisfaction, stress, and recognition in a pediatric setting. *Pediatric Nursing, 30*(3), 219–227.

Freudenberger, H. J. (1974). Staff burn-out. *Journal of Social Issues, 30*(1), 159–165. doi:10.1111/j.1540-4560.1974.tb00706.x

Golembiewski, R. T., Boudreau, R. A., Munzenrider, R. F., & Luo, H. (1996). *Global burnout: A world-wide pandemic explored by the phase model.* Greenwich, CT: JAI Press.

Goodman, S. (2007). Piercing the veil: The marginalization of midwives in the United States. *Social Sciences & Medicine, 65*(3), 610–621.

Gustaffson, G., Eriksson, S., Strandberg, G., & Norberg, A. (2010). Burnout and perceptions of conscience among health care personnel: A pilot study. *Nursing Ethics, 17*(1), 23–38. doi:10.1177/0969733009351950

Maslach, C., & Jackson, S. E. (1981). *The Maslach Burnout Inventory.* Palo Alto, CA: Consulting Psychologists Press.

Maslach, C., & Jackson, S. E. (1986). *Maslach Burnout Inventory manual* (2nd ed.). Palo Alto, CA: Consulting Psychologists Press.

Maslach, C., Jackson, S. E., & Leiter, M. P. (1997). Maslach burnout inventory. In C. P. Zalaquett & R. J. Woods (Eds.), *Evaluating stress: A book of resources* (3rd ed., pp. 191–218). Lanham, MD: Scarecrow Press.

Maslach, C., & Leiter, M. P. (2005). Stress and burnout: The critical research. In C. L. Cooper (Ed.), *Handbook of stress medicine and health* (2nd ed., pp. 143–170). London, England: CRC Press.

Maslach, C., & Leiter, M. P. (2008). Early predictors of job burnout and engagement. *Journal of Applied Psychology, 93*(3), 498–512. doi:10.1037/0021-9010.93.3.498

Pennsylvania Department of Health. (2011). *Pennsylvania vital statistics, 2008.* Retrieved from http://www.portal.state.pa.us/portal/server.pt?open=514&objID=596032& mode=2

Pennsylvania State Board of Medicine. (2011). *Licensure information.* Retrieved from http://www.portal.state.pa.us/portal/server.pt/community/state_board_of_ medicine/12512/licensure_information/599413

Rosenberg, T., & Pace, M. (2006). Burnout among mental health professionals: Special considerations for the marriage and family therapist. *Journal of Marital and Family Therapy, 32*(1), 87–99. doi:10.1111/j.1752-0606.2006.tb01590.x

Schaufeli, W. B., & Bakker, A. B. (2004). Job demands, job resources, and their relationship with burnout and engagement: A multi-sample study. *Journal of Organizational Behavior, 25*(3), 293–315. doi:10.1002/job.248

Schaufeli, W. B., & Buunk, B. P. (2003). Burnout: An overview of 25 years of research and theorizing. In M. J. Schabracq, J. A. Winnubst, & C. L. Cooper (Eds.), *The handbook of work and health psychology* (pp. 383–425). Chichester, England: Wiley.

Schaufeli, W. B., Leiter, M. P., & Maslach, C. (2009). Burnout: 35 years of research and practice. *Career Development International, 14*(3), 204–220. doi:10.1108/13620430910966406

Turnipseed, D. L. (1998). Anxiety and burnout in the health care work environment. *Psychological Reports, 82*(2), 627–642. doi:10.2466/pr0.1998.82.2.627

Vahey, D. C., Aiken, L. H., Sloane, D. M., Clarke, S. P., & Vargas, D. (2004). Nurse burnout and patient satisfaction. *Medical Care, 42*(Suppl. 2), 57–66. doi:10.1097/01.mlr .0000109126.503

Worley, J. A., Vassar, M., Wheeler, D. L., & Barnes, L. L. (2008). Factor structure of scores from the Maslach Burnout Inventory: A review and meta-analysis of 45 exploratory and confirmatory factor-analysis studies. *Educational and Psychological Measurement, 68*(5), 797–823. doi:10.1177/0013164408315268

5

Changing the Paradigm: Diabetic Group Visits in a Primary Care Setting

Gwendolyn Short

DNP Essential #2

Organizational and systems leadership for quality improvement and systems thinking

American Association of Colleges of Nursing. (2006). *The essentials of doctoral education for advanced nursing practice.* Retrieved from http://www.aacn.nche.edu/publications/position/DNPEssentials.pdf

This chapter describes a systems-level change in implementing diabetic group visits in a primary care clinic staffed by family practice residents.

It exemplifies DNP *Essential #2* as it relates to using systems thinking to improve the quality of health care.

Barbara A. Anderson, Editor

CAPSTONE FOCUS

The purpose of this project was to assess the impact of introducing the Chronic Care Model, and specifically one component of that model, group visits, on the delivery of health care to diabetic patients in a family medicine clinic and residency training program. The focus of this project was one component of an ongoing, national collaborative, the Academic Chronic Care Collaborative (ACCC), which included the project site as one of its 22 institutional member teams (Baxley & Stanek, 2007). The goal of this larger collaborative, the ACCC, was to improve care of patients with chronic illness and the educational outcomes of health professional students in the delivery of care to the chronically ill (Baxley & Stanek, 2007; Improving Chronic Illness Care, 2014).

The group visit is one available strategy to attempt improvements in redesigning the delivery of health care delivery services. The health care delivery system is one of the six Chronic Care Model (CCM) components that can be targeted for change. The scope of this project was to measure patient perceptions of their health care and changes in specific diabetes clinical indicators as a result of attendance at the diabetic group visits.

REVIEW OF THE LITERATURE

Chronic conditions are the leading cause of illness in the United States, consuming a major portion of U.S. health care resources (Institute of Medicine [IOM], 2001). Seven of ten deaths among Americans every year are due to chronic diseases (Centers for Disease Control and Prevention [CDC], 2014a). The medical care costs of people with chronic diseases account for more than 75% of the nation's $1.4 trillion medical care costs (Centers for Medicare and Medicaid Services [CMS], 2014). Chronic conditions often lead to debilitating health, since symptoms of the conditions go untreated, leaving patients with distressing symptoms that impact their quality of life (IOM, 2001; CDC, 2014a).

Diabetes is of particular concern because of its epidemic status. Through prevalence data gathered by the National Diabetes Surveillance System (NDSS), the CDC's estimated diabetes prevalence in the United States in adults aged 20 years or older in 2010 was 25.8 million, or 11.3% of the population in this age group, and 8.5% of the total U.S. population. More than seven million of these people do not know they have diabetes (CDC, 2014b). Estimates of individuals with undiagnosed diabetes are based on applying prevalence survey data of various civilian, noninstitutionalized population groups and applying it to the 2010 population (CDC, 2014b). Prediabetes is estimated to affect another 79 million Americans aged 20 and older (CDC, 2014b).

Complications of diabetes include heart disease, high blood pressure, stroke, kidney disease, blindness, and neuropathy. Adults with diabetes have heart disease death rates two to four times higher than adults without diabetes, while the risk of stroke is two to four times higher for those with diabetes. Heart disease and stroke account for approximately 65% of all deaths in people with diabetes (CDC, 2014b).

The prevalence of diabetes in Kentucky in 2010 was greater than that in the United States—10.4% in Kentucky versus 8.5% in the United States (Kentucky Cabinet for Health and Family Services, 2014). Kentucky ranks fourth among all states in diabetes prevalence, and based on estimates approximately 370,000 adult Kentuckians had a diagnosis of diabetes in 2010 (Kentucky Cabinet for Health and Family Services, 2014).

Challenges to Health Care Providers and Educators

In the 7 years since this capstone project was completed, more attention has been focused on the improvement of care processes in the clinical setting. This has been greatly facilitated by the introduction of the electronic health record across all clinical arenas. However, at the time of this project, the evidence was clear that clinical care processes did not reflect the scientific evidence of best care practices.

The Institute of Medicine (2001) described the dilemma of health care quality in the United States as a "quality chasm," the difference between what is considered evidence-based appropriate care and the usual care that is actually provided. Health care providers are challenged to provide ongoing patient management; deliver and coordinate care across teams, settings, and timeframes; and to support a patient's attempt to change behaviors and lifestyles (IOM, 2003). This is a daunting task, and one not being done well.

McGlynn and colleagues (2003) studied the extent to which standard processes of care for 30 selected acute, chronic, and preventive services were performed by health care providers in 12 U.S. metropolitan areas. This study included care received at a variety of health care settings, including inpatient and primary care facilities. Their findings indicated that, on average, Americans received about half of recommended medical care processes (acute, 53.5%; chronic, 56.1%; preventive, 54.9%). Thirteen processes of care for diabetes were measured, and found to be performed on an average of 45.4% of the time. These data clearly indicate that care processes need improvement.

Steinberg (2003) outlined a systematic approach to quality improvement and argued for: (1) consistent measurement and reporting of care, at both national and provider-specific levels; (2) improved and increased use of technology, especially point-of-care decision support tools; (3) meaningful involvement of patients in their health and health care; and (4) readjustment of current financial incentives to encourage quality improvement efforts.

Chronic Illness in Medical Education

Most leaders in medical education agree that academic health centers and medical schools need to make quality improvement more prominent in their curricula. Because chronic illnesses are among the most prevalent, costly, and preventable of all health problems (CDC, 2014a), it is imperative that quality improvement efforts pay particular attention to improving chronic illness care. Recognizing this need, the Association of American Medical Colleges (AAMC), in collaboration with the Robert Wood Johnson Foundation and 22 educational institutions, launched the ACCC in 2005. Using a systems-level approach, the 22 participating educational institutions, comprising 48 teams, began an extensive redesign of their chronic care strategies as well as provider education to integrate the CCM into practice (Baxley & Stanek, 2007).

The Chronic Care Model (CCM)

The CCM is a conceptual model to help guide improvement in chronic illness care (Coleman, Austin, Brach, & Wagner, 2009). Proposed as a model to help guide the delivery of health to individuals with chronic illnesses in the primary care setting, the CCM considers four levels of operation (or intervention): the entire community, with its resources and public and private policies; the health

FIGURE 5.1 *Overview of the Chronic Care Model*

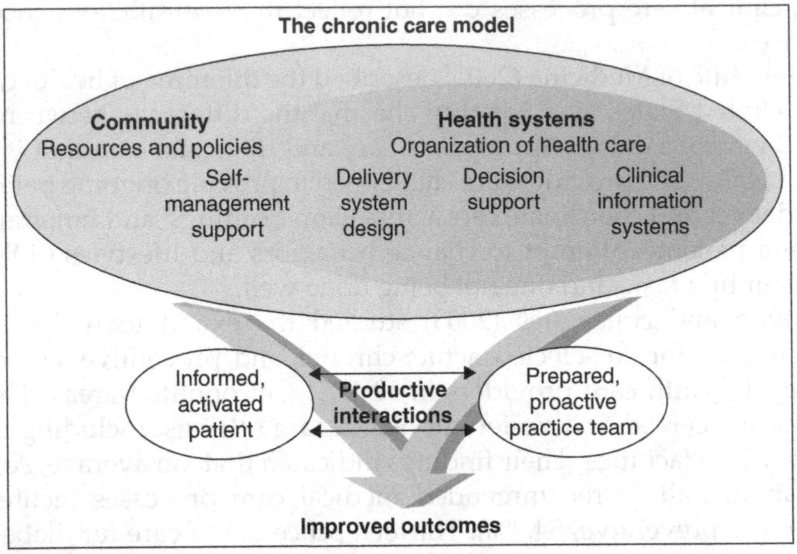

The chronic care model

Community
Resources and policies

Health systems
Organization of health care

Self-
management
support

Delivery
system
design

Decision
support

Clinical
information
systems

Informed,
activated
patient

**Productive
interactions**

Prepared,
proactive
practice team

Improved outcomes

Source: Improving Chronic Illness Care (2014).

care system, including its payment structures; the provider organization, which could be an integrated delivery system, a small clinic, or a loose network of physician practices; and the individual patient (see Figure 5.1).

Improving Chronic Illness Care (ICIC), a national program of the Robert Wood Johnson Foundation, employs the CCM as its conceptual framework to: promote effective change in health plans and provider groups; foster regional improvement initiatives; create and distribute resources and link innovators nationwide; and advance rigorous research in chronic care innovations (ICIC, 2014). Using the CCM as its framework, the ACCC is an example of a collaborative strategy to impact system change within academic institutions and associated care clinics.

Group Visits

Group visits, originally developed for use in the field of mental health, fall within the CCM component of "delivery system design." In the mid-1990s, psychologist Noffsinger (1999) adapted the group visit concept to deliver care to patients with chronic illnesses at Kaiser Permanente Medical Center in San Jose, California. This model of care, called the Drop-in Group Medical Appointment (DIGMA), consists of an extended medical appointment, custom-designed around the specific needs, goals, practice style, and patient panel constituency of the individual physician (Noffsinger & Scott, 2000). Another model of group visit care, the Cooperative Health Care Clinic (CHCC), focuses on the management of patients with specific high-risk diseases, such as diabetes, heart failure, depression, and asthma. Both models are expected to play an increasingly important role in the future delivery of health care (Noffsinger & Scott, 2000).

The core characteristic of a group visit is the delivery of medical care in a group setting with other patients. Specific advantages to this type of visit include increased time with the health care provider, a relaxed pace of care, improved efficiency and productivity, closer follow-up care, a more holistic approach, and information and support provided by other patients (Noffsinger & Scott, 2000).

THE CAPSTONE PROJECT

The site for this project was the University of Kentucky Department of Family and Community Medicine, Family Medicine Clinic (FMC), with its affiliated clinic and residency-training program, in collaboration with the Colleges of Nursing and Pharmacy. The author, a DNP student, worked as a family nurse practitioner at this clinic, as part of her academic appointment at the University of Kentucky's College of Nursing. The target patient population consisted of 625 patients who had a diagnosis of diabetes and who received their primary health care through the FMC. The project population reflected the clinic patient population:

- Age—18 and older
- Gender—men and women
- Ethnicity—all races (primarily Caucasian and African American)
- Anticipated number—maximum of 100

The FMC was chosen as the site for this project because of its participation in the University of Kentucky ACCC (UKACCC).

Project Implementation

This was a pilot quality improvement project to evaluate the impact of group visits on patient satisfaction and clinical outcomes of patients with diabetes. The primary objectives of this project were to evaluate (a) perception of care among patients with diabetes who attended the group visits, and (b) clinical outcomes, using seven specific diabetes care indicators. These seven indicators included having:

- A self-management goal
- Hemoglobin A1c less than 7%
- Blood pressure less than 130/80
- A comprehensive foot exam within the past year
- Been placed on a blood pressure medication that protects the kidneys (angiotensin-converting enzyme inhibitors [ACE] or angiotensin II receptor blockers [ARB])
- Received the influenza vaccine
- Been prescribed aspirin or other antithrombotic agent

Group visit participants were identified through verbal interaction with clinic staff and through identification of diagnosis as charted in the patient medical record. Participants were recruited by:

- A flyer posted in the FMC waiting room describing the project (Appendix A)

■ Verbal invitation by a health care provider or staff member during a regular clinic visit

■ Verbal invitation by a triage nurse during telephone interaction

The project coordinator was one of 20 providers at the FMC, and followed the same recruiting procedure as all other providers and clinic staff. Health care providers (a combination of nurses, faculty physicians, resident physicians, clinical support staff, nurse practitioners, nurse practitioner students, pharmacists, and physician's assistants) were present at various group visits. Invitation to participate in the group visits clearly stated that the participants were invited to take part in a research project about the group visits, but could participate in the visits without consenting to participate in the research.

Team members began to develop a registry of FMC patients with diabetes. Electronic health records were not yet available in the FMC, so the project coordinator reviewed paper health records. DocSite, described as a tool to assist with patient planning and point-of-care decision making, has been used in the development of the diabetic patient registry, beginning with those patients who participated in the diabetic group visit project (Millard, 2010). The DocSite's Patient Planner component, which specifically targets chronic disease management, was used to customize needs of the FMC project in data collection and tracking.

Meetings were held with representatives of the clinic's billing agency to ensure that appropriate coding and documentation were completed following the group visits. Group visits were a new concept to the billing and compliance offices, so administrative policies and procedures had not yet been developed to adequately deal with the billing and reimbursement activities surrounding the group visit.

Adjustments were made in the billing codes to be used. A group visit form was developed and revised to include in the patient record to document the care provided during the group visit. This information included clinical data, education received, problems identified, action taken, and referrals made. The format for the 90-minute visit included introduction (10 minutes); presentation of planned educational topics (20 minutes); discussion/question and answer (20 minutes); wrap-up (10 minutes); and 1:1 time with the health care provider (30 minutes). Educational topics presented at five monthly sessions included foot care, nutrition, medication management, exercise and diabetes care, and tips on taking care of your diabetes.

Measurement Instruments

Data collected consisted of survey and interview data, chart review, and measurable clinical data. The patient survey and interview data were obtained through use of the Patient Assessment of Chronic Illness Care (PACIC), a validated questionnaire developed by the Institute for Chronic Illness Care (www .improvingchroniccare.org). This tool, developed for use with the CCM, measures the extent to which patients with chronic illness receive care that aligns with the CCM, measuring care that is patient-centered, proactive, and planned and includes collaborative goal setting, problem-solving, and follow-up support.

Patients were asked to complete the PACIC at the end of their first visit or return it by mail. Participants were also asked to complete the PACIC at the end of the project. Use of the PACIC was not the standard care at the time of the project and was the only data collection measure in the project not a component of standard clinical care.

Findings

Participants were requested to complete the PACIC survey during their first group visit and again at the end of the project. Thirteen of 20 group visit participants completed the initial survey, a response rate of 65%. Because the group visits were temporarily discontinued before the final group visit was held, there was no opportunity for participants to complete the final survey during a group visit. The author mailed the second and final survey to the same 20 participants, and received a return of nine surveys, a response rate of 45%. Analysis of survey results indicates a 34% overall improvement score in patient perception of their care. Improvement was seen in 25 of the 26 measures, seven of which showed improvement by at least 50% (see Table 5.1).

Respondents to the pre- and postsurveys were not identified, and in all likelihood were not the same in both groups. A summary score was obtained

TABLE 5.1 *PACIC Data Showing Improvement > 50%*

	Presurvey Scores (n = 13)	Postsurvey Scores (n = 9)	Percentage Change
Asked for my ideas when we made a treatment plan.	3	4.6	+ 53
Given choices about treatment to think about.	2.8	4.4	+ 57
Helped to set specific goals to improve my eating or exercise.	3	4.6	+ 53
Given a copy of my treatment plan.	2.3	4	+ 74
Encouraged to go to a specific group or class to help me cope with my chronic illness.	2.8	4.3	+ 54
Helped to plan ahead so I could take care of my illness even in hard times.	2.6	4	+ 54
Set a goal together with my team for what I could do to manage my condition.	2.7	4.3	+ 59

of pre- and postsurvey results, and Statistical Package for the Social Sciences (SPSS) software was used to perform an independent *t*-test to compare the mean scores. There was not a statistical significance between the pre- and postsurvey scores ($t = -1.785$). A decline in scores was seen in one of the questions: measuring how the primary care providers inform patients on the role of specialist referrals in their treatment.

Clinical indicator measures were retrieved through a health record review at the beginning and end of the project. Data included health information that had been entered into the medical record October 1, 2005 through July 31, 2006. The seven clinical indicators measured for this project were identical to those chosen by the University of Kentucky (UK) team to track its participation in the ACCC. Four of the measures were mandated by the ACCC, including self-management goal, HA1c < 7%, BP < 130/70, and comprehensive foot exam within the past year. The remaining three measures were chosen by the UKACCC team as additional measures. These included whether patients were placed on an ACE or ARB (kidney-protecting antihypertensive agent), evaluated for beginning aspirin or another antithrombotic agent, and having received an influenza vaccine within the past year. Table 5.2 compares these measures before and after the group visit project.

The data indicate improvement in six of the seven measures, with the blood pressure measure showing no change. SPSS was used to determine the Pearson Chi-Square value for each indicator. Statistical significance was seen in four of seven measures at the 0.05 significance level.

TABLE 5.2 *Clinical Measurements at the Beginning and End of a Group Visit Project*

Measure	First Visit n (%)	Last Visit n (%)	% Change	Chi-Square (p)
Has self-management goal	3/19 (16%)	9/19 (47%)	31%	4.385 (.036)
HbAlc < 7%	7/20 (35%)	10/20 (50%)	15%	0.925 (.337)
BP < 130/70	7/20 (35%)	7/20 (35%)	0	0.0 (1.0)
Has received comprehensive foot exam in past year	7/20 (35%)	17/20 (85%)	50%	10.417 (.001)
On ACE or ARB	4/20 (20%)	17/20 (85%)	75%	16.942 (< .001)
Has received influenza vaccine in past year	6/20 (30%)	7/20 (35%)	5%	0.051 (.821)
On ASA or other antithrombotic medications	4/19 (21%)	15/19 (79%)	58%	11.906 (.001)

Note: Missing data are due to missing health information in the medical record or unavailability of the record at time of review.

ACE = angiotensin-converting enzyme inhibitor; ARB = angiotensin II receptor blockers; ASA = acetylsalicylic acid.

PROJECT IMPACT

While improvement in the PACIC scores and diabetes clinical indicators showed a positive impact on both patient perception of care and clinical outcomes, the most important impact of this project was on the various system components of the health care environment. One of these components was the family medicine residency education program within the academic health center, which, at the end of the project, adopted the CCM as a framework to use in the department's redesign of its residency education program aimed at improving strategies for teaching chronic illness care.

A problematic financial issue that became apparent during the course of this project was the process surrounding billing for reimbursement of the group visits. Several UKACCC team members met with the clinic's billing agency during project planning stages. The billing agent had never been asked to submit claims for this type of service, but a review of billing regulations indicated an appropriate code describing group education. This code was used to reflect the charges for the group visit activities for each participant. Medicare, however, refused payment on these claims because of specific guidelines in place for group activities that relate to diabetes education. Other ACCC member institutions were queried, and the majority of those conducting and billing for group visits used an "Evaluation and Management" (E&M) code, with billing submitted under a single provider name. The UK compliance office decided that an E&M code did not accurately reflect the care provided during a group visit, so if used could be viewed as a fraudulent billing claim by Medicare. A phone call to the regional Medicare office supported this decision. Determinations of Medicare payment differed nationally between regions.

One effective impact of the diabetic group visit project on technology was the decision to have the FMC serve as a test site for expansion of the University of Kentucky Hospital's EHR into the ambulatory care arena. The goal for this was to provide important process and outcome data for further implementation of EHR into the university's outpatient setting. FMC faculty were queried as to their readiness to participate in this process, and with a few exceptions, the overall response was enthusiastic.

A significant change in communication processes occurred over the course of this project. Planning and initiating the group visits created changes in communication behaviors between individuals and institutional departments. ACCC team members represented parts of the FMC that did not normally work together, for example, the medical educator and the nurse practitioner. Similarly, because group visits were a new concept within the institution, developing an appropriate guideline for documentation and choosing an appropriate code for reimbursement required team members to meet and problem solve with staff from the institution's billing office. These types of interdisciplinary and interdepartmental work activities created opportunities for creative thinking and problem solving.

CONCLUSION

In the 8 years since implementation of this DNP capstone project, there have been many changes in health care impacting all levels, including the nation, communities, institutions, and individuals. The author is no longer at the Family

Medical Center. The diabetic group visits continued for several months follow-ing the project completion, but were forced to end because the reimbursement issue never got settled, and were financially unsustainable. Due to the federal mandate, the UK clinic system has since developed an electronic health record, easing the way for development of patient registries for all types of illnesses, not just diabetes. The CCM continues to serve as a foundation for teaching the family medical residents how to care for patients with chronic illnesses and is a working conceptual guide for clinical quality improvement efforts (E. Tovar, personal communication, January 21, 2014). The group visit capstone project can be credited, in part, for initiating some early cultural, clinical processes, and educational changes within the FMC.

The CCM has continued to grow and expand, developing innovative frame-works to support clinical improvement within regional health care systems, includ-ing home care services, while supporting the concepts of the patient-centered medical home and team care (ICIC, 2014). Evaluation studies of the effective-ness of the CCM have been mixed. While it appears as if the CCM provides a conceptual framework to guide practice redesign, leading to improved patient care and better health outcomes (Coleman, Austin, Brach, & Wagner, 2009), the model has also been criticized as being too broad to guide implementation of the model's change processes (Hroscikoski et al., 2006; Solberg et al., 2006).

On a final note, a qualitative study of the CCM implementation in a large health system in Minnesota demonstrated a need for more prescriptive change strategies than provided by the model (Hroscikoski et al., 2006). Physicians in this study were not engaged in a meaningful way with the clinical change process. The authors of this study concluded that this was due to the tradition and orga-nizational history of physician autonomy (Hroscikoski et al., 2006). In contrast, the roles of the nurses and clerical staff changed the most, with nurses becoming the change agents, performing case management activities, and clerical workers becoming more directly involved with the patients. This is similar to what the author found as a result of her own DNP capstone implementation projection.

Use of the CCM is a good fit with the work done by both nurses and nurse practitioners. With knowledge of patient advocacy, patient-centered interview-ing, team-based care, holistic health care, and patient management, nurses and nurse practitioners have an excellent understanding of this model. The author noticed this immediately during the participant training sessions provided by the ACCC where sessions were held on motivational interviewing, patient-centered health care, and registry development. Nurse team members easily performed the learning activities during these learning sessions. Such collab-orative care can improve care processes and patient outcomes. A remaining barrier is the hierarchical structures of most health care systems.

REFERENCES

Baxley, E. G., & Stanek, M. (2007). The AAMC academic chronic care collaborative: Fam-ily medicine's participation and lessons learned. *Annals of Family Medicine, 5*(2), 183–184. doi:10.1370/afm.688

Centers for Medicare and Medicaid Services. (2014). *National health expenditures 2012 highlights*. Retrieved from http://www.cms.gov/NationalHealthExpendData

Centers for Disease Control and Prevention. (2014a). *Chronic diseases and health promotion*. Retrieved from http://www.cdc.gov/chronicdisease/overview/index.htm#1

Centers for Disease Control and Prevention. (2014b). *National diabetes fact sheet, 2011*. Retrieved from http://www.cdc.gov/diabetes/pubs/pdf/ndfs_2011.pdf

Coleman, K., Austin, B. T., Brach, C., & Wagner, E. H. (2009). Evidence on the chronic care model in the new millennium. *Health Affairs, 28*(1), 75–85. doi:10.1377/hlthaff.28.1.75

Hroscikoski, M. C., Solberg, L. I., Sperl-Hillen, J. M., Harper, P. G., McGrail, M. P., & Crabtree, B. F. (2006). Challenges of change: A qualitative study of Chronic Care Model implementation. *Annals of Family Medicine, 4*(4), 317–326. doi:10.1370/afm.570

Improving Chronic Illness Care. (2014). *Patient-centered medical home*. Retrieved from http://improvingchroniccare.org/index.php?p=Patient-Centered_Medical_Home&s=224

Institute of Medicine. (2001). *Crossing the quality chasm: A new health system for the 21st century*. Washington, DC: Institute of Medicine, The National Academies Press. Retrieved from http://www.iom.edu/Reports/2001/Crossing-the-Quality-Chasm-A-New-Health-System-for-the-21st-Century.aspx

Institute of Medicine. (2003). *Health professions education: A bridge to quality*. Washington: Institute of Medicine, The National Academies Press. doi:10.1177/152715440325830 Available from http://www.nap.edu/catalog.php?record_id=10681

Kentucky Cabinet for Health and Family Services. (2014). *General information about diabetes*. Retrieved from http://chfs.ky.gov/dph/info/dpqi/cd/generalinfodiabetes.htm

McGlynn, E. A., Asch, S. M., Adams, J., Keesey, J., Hicks, J., DeCristofaro, A., & Kerr, E. A. (2003). The quality of health care delivered to adults in the United States. *The New England Journal of Medicine, 248*(26), 2635–2645.

Millard, M. (2010). Covisint acquires DocSite. *Healthcare IT News*. Retrieved from http://www.healthcareitnews.com/news/covisint-acquires-docsite-0

Noffsinger, E. B. (1999). Increasing quality of care and access while reducing costs through drop-in group medical appointments (DIGMAs). *Group Practice Journal, 48(1)*, 12–18.

Noffsinger, E. B., & Scott, J. C. (2000). Preventing potential abuses of group visits. *Group Practice Journal, 49*(5), 37–48.

Solberg, L. I., Crain, A. L., Sperl-Hillen, J. M., Hroscikoski, M. C., Engebretson, K. I., & O'Connor, P. J. (2006). Care quality and implementation of the Chronic Care Model: A quantitative study. *Annals of Family Medicine, 4*(4), 310–316. doi:10.1370/afm.571

Steinberg, E. P. (2003). Improving the quality of care—Can we practice what we preach? *New England Journal of Medicine, 348*(26), 2681–2683.

6

Promoting Compassion Fatigue Resiliency Among Emergency Department Nurses

Kathleen Flarity, Elizabeth Holcomb, and J. Eric Gentry

DNP Essential #3

Clinical scholarship and analytical methods for evidence-based practice

American Association of Colleges of Nursing. (2006). *The essentials of doctoral education for advanced nursing practice.* Retrieved from http://www.aacn.nche.edu/publications/position/DNPEssentials.pdf

This chapter describes the development of a training program for emergency nurses to prevent compassion fatigue and strengthen resiliency skills in a high acuity setting.

It exemplifies DNP *Essential #3* as it relates to using clinical scholarship and analytical methods to develop an evidence-based program targeting a major mental health risk for emergency nurses.

Barbara A. Anderson, Editor

CAPSTONE FOCUS

Emergency nurses work in an environment that is intellectually, emotionally, and physically demanding with repetitive exposure to the stressors of the emergency department (ED), which includes chaos, overcrowding, high patient acuity, workplace violence, prolonged patient holding, unrealistic patient expectations, trauma, and death. Compassion fatigue (CF) may result. It is a significant issue among health care providers as they bring more than skill and knowledge to their jobs. They also bring empathy and quality of caregiving in their relationships with their patients (Flarity, Gentry, & Mesnikoff, 2013). This capstone project focused on the prevention of CF and the promotion of resiliency among emergency department nurses.

REVIEW OF THE LITERATURE

Caregiving takes an emotional, physical, professional, spiritual, and relational toll upon health care providers (Dominguez-Gomez & Rutledge, 2009; Figley, 2002a, 2002b; Flarity, 2011; Flarity et al., 2013; Gentry, 2002; Roney, 2010; Strommer, 2011). The first author (KF) has witnessed the impact of this toll in both her civilian and military experiences. She has seen colleagues suffer and leave the health professions as a result.

Compassion Fatigue (CF)

The adverse psychological impact on care providers has been described under a variety of terms, including caregiver stress, vicarious traumatization, countertransference, secondary traumatic stress (STS), burnout (BO), posttraumatic stress disorder (PTSD), and CF (Figley, 1995, 2002a). Figley (1995) describes CF as a "... state of exhaustion and dysfunction (biological, psychological and social) as a result of prolonged exposure to compassion stress" (p. 15), characterized by two components: BO and STS.

BO is a form of job stress with chronic emotional overload (Figley, 1995). It is the result of work-related factors including high patient acuity, workplace violence, understaffing, prolonged patient holding, overcrowding, unrealistic scheduling, high patient expectations, and lack of support from leadership. BO encompasses feelings of exhaustion, frustration, anger, hopelessness, feeling overwhelmed, depression, and a sense that one's work makes no difference (Gentry, 2012; Stamm, 2009). Gentry (2012) attributes the symptoms of BO to the perception that demands outweigh resources.

The corollary, STS, is the negative effects of witnessing trauma, pain, and suffering (Gentry, 2002, 2012; Stamm, 2009). The cumulative effects of exposure to the distress and suffering of others may lead to CF symptomatology such as intrusive thoughts, physical symptoms, avoidance behaviors, sleep disturbances, and hyperarousal (Flarity et al., 2013). These symptoms may interfere with the ability to cope with the stresses involved in providing care (Figley, 1995, 2002b, 2007; Flarity et al., 2013; Huggard, 2003; Laposa, Alden & Fullerton, 2003). Repeated exposure to STS can have a negative cumulative effect (Gentry, 2012; Pearlman & Saakvitne, 1995).

There are a few small studies indicating that emergency department nurses are at risk for CF, but the prevalence of CF in these nurses is unknown (Dominguez-Gomez & Rutledge, 2009; Hooper, Craig, Janvrin, Wetsel, & Reimels, 2010). CF, while originally emerging from the field of traumatology, has been studied more widely in psychology, social work, and counseling (Figley & Kebler, 1995; Gentry, 2012). The diagnosis of CF is not recognized by the *Diagnostic and Statistical Manual of Mental Disorders, Fifth Edition* (*DSM-5*) (American Psychiatric Association [APA], 2013); however, *adjustment disorder with mixed emotional features* may be used as an alternative diagnosis for those suffering from CF (Flarity et al., 2013; Gentry, 2012). Usually CF is a self-identified diagnosis. However, many who are suffering from CF are not aware that they have it. The symptoms identified in patients with PSTD, such as intrusive thoughts, sleep disturbances, avoidance behaviors, anxiety, distressing emotions, physical ailments, and hyperarousal, are also present in some individuals with CF (Figley, 2002; Gentry, 2012; Stewart, 2009).

The Impact of Stress on the Nervous System

In high-stress environments, even without fear of physical harm, it is natural to experience sympathetic nervous system (SNS) activation (the fight or flight response). The person is not able to differentiate between a real threat (a tiger threatening to attack) and a perceived threat (trauma code). An empathetic human response combined with SNS arousal can result in escalating stress. For example, when hearing the whirl of helicopter blades or the siren of an ambulance, the health care provider may experience increased heart rate and blood pressure, rapid breathing, and sweaty palms as the brain and body go into SNS arousal. The biological basis for this stress has two sources: innate human empathy, and the physiological response arising from the caregiver role. Since most humans are deeply impacted by the suffering and pain of others, the repeated experience of caring for patients' suffering is one of the primary contributors to CF (Flarity et al., 2013).

Empathy is an innate human characteristic and there is "wiring" in the brain that creates empathic responses and, in some cases, the subsequent deleterious effects of CF. In a study of Macaque monkeys, researchers discovered that certain areas of the brain were activated not only while eating or drinking but also when merely observing other monkeys eating or drinking. Research with humans has found that similar areas in the brain, "mirror neurons," are stimulated by observation of a behavior (Rizzolatti & Fabbri-Destro, 2010). A number of studies have suggested that the mirror neuron system, at least in part, allows for human empathic responses (Flarity et al., 2013).

The empathetic health care provider, with responsibility to alleviate suffering, may experience CF, an exaggerated physiological response and heightened SNS arousal, similar to PTSD. PTSD was first recognized as a psychological war wound among soldiers (Stewart, 2009). Victims of PTSD can typically recall the event(s) that trigger PTSD symptoms such as a gunshot wound, a traumatic amputation, or rape; CF is more insidious and often unrecognized, yet it can be just as life altering (Flarity et al., 2013; Stewart, 2009). Figley (2002b) describes CF as "nearly identical to PTSD, except that it applies to those emotionally affected by the trauma of another" (p. 3).

The Impact of Culture on Compassion Fatigue

In addition, a job culture that indirectly or openly encourages staff members to be emotionally tough may exacerbate the stressors and further predispose or accelerate the progression of CF. This culture may also result in reluctance to seek help (Flarity et al., 2013).

And furthermore,

> Burned-out physicians and nurses are often reluctant to seek help, seeing such a request as a threat to the public's, and their own, confidence in their ability and self-image. Emergency department staff will usually respond to BO by working at their usual level or even harder when good sense and judgment indicate otherwise. (Phipps, 1998, p. 375)

Programs to Combat Compassion Fatigue

All health care professionals are at risk for CF, and seeking support should be encouraged and regarded as normal rather than a weakness (Flarity et al., 2013; Gentry, 2012). In 1997, Gentry, Baranowsky, and Dunning, under the direction of renowned traumatologist Charles Figley, developed the first comprehensive treatment program for CF. This five-session Accelerated Recovery Program (ARP) for CF combines several trauma protocols, a comprehensive assessment, and a self-administered self-care plan (Gentry, 2002; Gentry, Baranowsky, & Dunning, 2002). Since 1997, Gentry has reported that the symptoms of CF are very responsive to ARP treatment. Coining the phrase "training as treatment," Gentry et al. (2002) notes that health care professionals who attended the ARP are able to help others as well as themselves.

In 1998, in response to the success of the ARP, Gentry and Baranowsky developed the Certified Compassion Fatigue Specialist Training (CCFST), a comprehensive training program to help professionals provide interventions for caregivers suffering from CF (Gentry et al., 2002). Gentry then introduced a packet of trainings: the Certified Compassion Fatigue Specialist Training, and the Compassion Fatigue Prevention and Resiliency Training. These two trainings have demonstrated treatment effectiveness for the symptoms of CF (Gentry et al., 2002).

Another approach is guided imagery. Naparastek (2006) reported that guided imagery has been highly effective among patients with PTSD. However, there was no guided imagery intervention specifically designed for or evaluated in emergency nurses. My personal experience (KF) as an aeromedical evacuation commander in Afghanistan supported the use of Naparastek's guided imagery for alleviating CF (Flarity et al., 2013).

These approaches teach psychological and physiological self-regulation of parasympathetic dominance, reducing SNS arousal, and creating an internal state where providers can be compassionate and connected to patients without taking on the trauma and suffering of others. These self-regulatory approaches support psychological sustainability in settings with frequent exposure to traumatic events as well as social and personal situations (Flarity et al., 2013). The goal of these programs is to achieve compassion satisfaction, ".... joy, purpose, and meaning care givers derive from their work" (Flarity et al., 2013, p. 249).

THE CAPSTONE PROJECT

Emergency nurses may need support to cope with the negative effects of their high-stress work (Figley, 2002b; Figley & Kebler, 1995; Gentry, 2012; Gentry et al., 2002; Gillespie, Gates & Succop, 2010; Naparastek, 2006; Pearlman & Saakvitne, 1995). Despite exposure to stress in their daily professional lives, there has been minimal study of the cumulative effects of this stress on emergency nurses (Dominguez-Gomez & Rutledge, 2009).

Prior to this DNP capstone, there were no published interventions on prevention of CF or programs to increase resiliency among emergency nurses. I (KF) wanted to learn more about both prevention and treatment of the problem. I studied to become a certified compassion fatigue specialist (CCFS) and I framed my doctoral capstone around this topic. Despite 33 years of working in civilian and military level 1 trauma centers and flight programs, I scored high on compassion satisfaction and low on the two components of CF: BO and STS. Even with my positive scores going into the CCFS training, I was impacted profoundly by the experience, both professionally and personally. I noted a positive change in myself and my impact on people around me. I experienced less stress and more joy, purpose, and meaning from my work and in my relationships.

Overview of the Capstone Project

The study sites were two emergency departments in Colorado with a combined 140,000 annual patient visits. I aimed to offer CF resiliency training to emergency care nurses at these sites. I envisioned that the spiritual services and behavioral health specialists would expand the program system wide, promoting sustainability.

My capstone committee was comprised of my chair, Dr. Elizabeth Holcomb, PhD, FNP, professor at Frontier Nursing University, whose clinical background includes flight nursing in Alaska and FNP services with the Army Reserves and National Guard soldiers recently returned from deployment. My content expert was Dr. J. Eric Gentry. In the implementation of this project, he offered the use of the tools he designed.

Study Design

A pre-/posttest design with participants serving as their own control group was used for this study. The convenience sample ($n = 73$) consisted of emergency nurses who self-selected to participate in the study by scheduling themselves for the multifaceted CF resiliency intervention program. Quantitative data were obtained from the Professional Quality of Life Tool (ProQOL; Stamm, 2009) and a demographic questionnaire (Flarity et al., 2013). The ProQOL is a 30-item self-report tool that uses three subscales: compassion satisfaction (CS), STS, and BO. The reliability and validity of the tool have been previously established, and it is the most widely used tool to measure the positive and negative aspects of caring (Gentry, 2002; Stamm, 2010). The ProQOL (version 5) by Stamm (2009) was employed as a pre-/posttest to examine the effectiveness of the multifaceted intervention on decreasing emergency nurses' CF and increasing compassion satisfaction.

Intervention

The first level of intervention was a 4-hour interactive group seminar entitled "Compassion Fatigue Resiliency" that I conducted with the spiritual services director. The seminar was adapted with permission from Gentry's (2012) *Compassion Fatigue Prevention and Resiliency: Fitness for the Frontline* course. The seminar began with a powerful documentary video about an aeromedical evacuation mission. The video is a professional documentary reenactment of the story described in the case study that follows.

CASE STUDY

The Art and Danger of Caring

As a deployed Air Force aeromedical evacuation (AE) commander in Afghanistan and an experienced emergency department nurse, I (KF) have witnessed countless friends and colleagues suffer from the effects of the work that they do. Military medical teams are highly skilled, educated professionals dedicated to their calling of caring for our nation's heroes. Military medical professionals are called to a mission of putting others first, service before self, and caring for America's sons, daughters, brothers, sisters, fathers, and mothers (Flarity, 2011).

Each day, as I saw American troops fighting and dying, I cared for the wounded and my heart ached for them and their families. However, I also empathized with the physicians, nurses, and technicians who cared for them. In the course of one AE mission, the airmen under my command often saw more than what most of humanity sees in a lifetime. The youth of the patients and the horrendous nature of the injuries take an emotional toll on military caregivers; "Legs without feet. Eyes that can't see. Brains that will never think the same again" (Vaughn, 2005, p. 1). It was not uncommon for one of the 19-year-old medics to care for a triple-amputee patient on an AE flight. The sights, sounds, intrusive thinking, avoidance behavior, and sleep disturbances may haunt the caregiver forever. My heart ached for them (Flarity, 2011).

After one of my deployments, a best friend, who had also been deployed, experienced considerable difficulty readjusting to life back home. He was detached at home and at work, his short temper and increased alcohol consumption was concerning to friends and family. He was an experienced emergency department nurse who worked in a Level 1 trauma facility. Providing care to trauma patients was not new to him. However, during his long AE missions providing care, he connected with his patients and heard the personal stories of the wounded warriors. He wrote the following story:

> The best way to describe his injuries is to say that chunks of his body are missing. He is in a lot of pain. He smells, is dirty, and has bandages that are leaking blood and serous fluid. The field hospital didn't have time to clean him up since he is a priority patient to evacuate. I've noticed that the most seriously injured are the youngest. The older, experienced soldiers do a better job of staying alive and avoiding the flying metal.
>
> The morphine is not working, but it's the strongest stuff I've got. I have to play a juggling act to keep my patient comfortable. At some point during

(continued)

(continued)

these adjustments I accidentally dislodge a Hemovac suction unit from one of his infected wounds. Foul-smelling, reddish-yellow fluid drains from the tube and drips off the litter. I start looking at his bandages to find the other end of the tubing. I open one bandage and find sand fleas where his toes used to be. I try my best to keep a straight face, but the sight of the fleas in his wound nauseates me. Steve, one of my level-headed medics, finds the tubing and resets the suction, then cleans up the mess I made.

We finally get this soldier comfortable. Because we moved him so much, I decide to reassess his extremities. The circulation is poor at the end of his legs, and what is left of his feet is swollen. I know there are parts of his leg and thigh missing from reading his medical record, but I can't tell from the thick bandages. The wounds were left open to allow them to drain. The dressings are wet and covered in a light layer of sand. I ask the soldier to wiggle the toes he has. We have direct eye contact. On one side his toes move fine; on the other side there is no movement. What is left on that side is cold and hard to touch. He looks at me and our eyes are locked. His eyes say, "Tell me I'm going to be O.K. Tell me that I'm going to be fine, tell me I'm going to be whole again. . ." These are some of the longest seconds of my life because I know he is counting on what I say to him. I bend down below the litter to break eye contact. I act like I'm adjusting some of the medical equipment attached to him. My mind is racing. I have always been honest with my patients. Do I lie or tell him the truth? The seconds move so slowly as I fight my internal battle on what is right. I stand straight up and there are his eyes. I'm at the end of the litter and with the noise of the plane there is no way he could hear me speak. We are now communicating solely with our eyes and facial expressions. The look on his face. . . the look. . . I felt like what I did next would determine his future. I'm sure less than 2 seconds passed before I gave him a big smile and a thumb's up. Those 2 seconds felt like an hour. He broke into a big smile of relief and I felt broken. (Hrivnak, 2013, p. 63)

Those last few words "and I felt broken" highlighted his anguish. Although this flight nurse, my friend and colleague, had no visible physical wounds, he was suffering his internal battle in caring for the wounded. He left the nursing profession and eventually, with urging, sought treatment. He was diagnosed with posttraumatic stress disorder (PTSD), although his presentation can also be described as CF.

While deployed in Afghanistan I received the message that my friend had died in the hospital parking lot where he worked. Although the autopsy report stated "self-inflicted gunshot wound to the head," we know a contributing cause of his death was CF. Caring for the traumatized, traumatizes (Figley, 2002b).

The remainder of the seminar used PowerPoint slides for an interactive lecture, group discussion, and group and individual exercises. The content included information about the origins of CF, the physiological effects, signs and symptoms of CF, as well as the factors associated with emergency nursing that may lead to CF. The seminar provided conceptual information and suggestions regarding prevention of and treatment for CF, including the five key elements identified for the prevention of and treatment of CF: self-regulation, intentionality, perceptual maturation/self-validated caregiving, connection, and self-care (Gentry, 2012).

In the second level of intervention, multimedia resources were provided or made available to the participants. The resources included:

■ Printed seminar handouts
■ "Tools of Hope" (Gentry, 2012)
■ Guided imaging (Naparastek, 2006)
■ Access to a website with CF, compassion satisfaction, and resiliency educational resources and publications (Gentry, 2012)

Data Analysis

Data were scored using the Statistical Package for the Social Sciences for the ProQOL and Microsoft Excel for demographics. Wilcoxon signed-rank tests were used to evaluate the differences. The level of significance of $p = 0.05$ was used for all tests for statistical significance (Flarity et al., 2013).

Evaluation

The participants ranged in experience from more than 20 years to 48 hours. In the pretest for this sample, the majority of participants ($n = 38$, 52%) had low to moderate levels of compassion satisfaction, and 43 participants (59%) reported moderate to high levels of BO, while 44 participants (60%) had moderate to high levels of STS. Forty-two participants (60%) reported at least one symptom of CF in the past 30 days.

Fifty-nine posttests were returned and included for analysis. The multifaceted education program showed statistical significance in increasing CS and in decreasing BO and STS symptoms (Table 6.1). The majority of the participants (61%) reported high levels of CS after the intervention. Twenty-nine participants (49%) reported low to moderate levels of CS on the pretest and only 23 (39%) reported low to moderate levels of compassion satisfaction on the posttest, indicating a 10% improvement after the intervention ($p = 0.004$) (Flarity et al., 2013).

For BO, 34 participants (58%) indicated moderate to high levels of BO in the pretest, and only 14 (24%) indicated moderate to high levels level of BO after the intervention, indicating a 34% improvement ($p = < 0.001$). In the pretest, 35 participants (59%) reported moderate to high levels of STS, but only 24 (41%) reported that level after the intervention, indicating a 19% improvement ($p = 0.001$).

The course evaluations subjectively indicated positive outcomes of the intervention. All of the participants rated the seminar as excellent, and all of the participants wrote positive comments on the evaluation form, such as: "The entire program was wonderful, uplifting, and self-validating; my inner confidence has increased and I am inspired"; "Such value in the material and its application to our lives and practice"; "Should be required"; "I now have compassion toward difficult people"; "Good for young nurses to prevent burnout"; and "I will apply the strategies to prevent/treat compassion fatigue" (Flarity et al., 2013).

TABLE 6.1 *Pre-/Posttest Comparison of Compassion Satisfaction, Burnout, and Secondary Traumatic Stress Scores*

Variable	Pretest n (%)	Posttest n (%)	Significance	Percent Improvement
Compassion Satisfaction (CS)				
High (good)	30 (50.8)	36 (61.0)	p = .004	10% reported
Moderate	28 (47.5)	23 (39.0)		higher compas-
Low (bad)	1 (1.7)	0		sion satisfaction
Burnout (BO)				
Low (good)	25 (42.4)	45 (76.3)	p < .001	34% reported
Moderate	33 (55.9)	14 (23.7)		lower burnout
High (bad)	1 (1.7)	0		symptoms
Secondary Traumatic Stress (STS)				
Low (good)	24 (40.7)	35 (59.3)	p = .001	19% reported
Moderate	34 (57.6)	24 (40.7)		lower secondary
High (bad)	1 (1.7)	0		traumatic stress
				symptoms

Source: Flarity et al. (2013).

IMPACT

The first author (KF) presented the results of *The Effectiveness of an Educational Program on Preventing and Treating Compassion Fatigue in Emergency Nurses* at a Colorado State Emergency Nurses Association meeting and a Trauma and Critical Care Symposium. She was also invited to present the *Compassion Fatigue Resiliency* seminar at the Colorado Forensic Nurse Examiners, the International Forensic Nurse Examiners Annual conference. The results of the study were presented at the Association of Military Surgeons of the United States conference. Additionally, since the study completion, the program has been presented in a 2-1/2 hour format to intensive care RNs and in-patient units. The results of this shortened version are pending.

Lastly, the manuscript, "The Effectiveness of an Educational Program on Preventing and Treating Compassion Fatigue in Emergency Nurses," was published in *The Advanced Emergency Nursing Journal* (August 2013). Sharing the study in these venues invites leaders and caregivers to consider their risk of CF and seek methods to prevent and treat CF in themselves and for their organizations. This program has demonstrated a low-cost, easy-to-implement method for enhancing CS and for diminishing the negative effects of work-related stress (BO and STS). It may prove to be valuable in academic and continuing education nursing educational programs.

CF can have an adverse effect on performance, morale, staff recruitment, and retention (Schwam, 1998). Emergency nurses with CF may no longer be effective with patients as their symptoms may interfere with providing empathetic care (Dominguez-Gomez & Rutledge, 2009). The cost to the nurse may be job stress, loss of promotion, job loss, or disruptive personal relations. The damage to the system may be suboptimal care, medication errors, poor compliance and follow-up from patients, and loss of referrals as a result of dissatisfaction with care. The national average cost of replacing an experienced nurse is estimated at $85,000 (American Organization of Nurse Executives [AONE], 2010). Although not measured in this study, a potential positive outcome of CS is retention of emergency nurses.

Challenging caregiving experiences affect not only the lives of emergency nurses, but also affect the lives of those who are close to them. Significant others, family members, friends, and colleagues may share in the negative effects of CF. On a personal and professional level, CF resiliency training has had a positive impact on my life (KF). In the course of my work as a caregiver and a military Commander, I am often exposed to the secondary traumatic stress of others and have witnessed the consequences of CF in friends and colleagues.

Through this project I have self-identified triggers that stimulate a sympathetic response at both home and work. Working toward parasympathetic dominance and control, I have been able to eliminate the response to some triggers. Simple things that used to be triggers, such as dishes in the sink, a traffic jam, a backfiring car (sounds like gunshots), or a challenging patient or colleague no longer affect me. I am now able to be fully present to engage in my life's calling and continue to receive joy, purpose, and meaning from my work.

CONCLUSION

All health care providers, by the nature of their work, are at risk for CF. However, CF prevention and resiliency is not addressed or taught in nursing education programs. As the first intervention study aiming to prevent and treat CF in emergency nurses, the results of this study have important implications. The findings of this capstone suggest that institutional programs may maximize caregivers' level of CS and reduce risks for developing CF. It exemplifies DNP *Essential #3: Clinical scholarship and analytical methods for evidence-based practice*, and exemplifies that "Our capacity to help others is greatest when we are willing and able and even determined to help ourselves" (van Dernoot Lipsky & Burk, 2009, p.19).

REFERENCES

American Organization of Nurse Executives. (2010). *AONE principles for the aging work-force*. Retrieved from http://www.aone.org/resources/PDFs/AONE_GP_Aging_Workforce.pdf

American Psychiatric Association. (2013). *Diagnostic and statistical manual of mental disorders*, fifth edition *(DSM-5)*. Retrieved from http://www.dsm5.org/about/Pages/DSMVOverview.aspx

Dominguez-Gomez, E., & Rutledge, D. N. (2009). Prevalence of secondary traumatic stress among emergency nurses. *Journal of Emergency Nursing, 35*(3), 199–204. doi:10.1016/j.jen.2008.05.003

Figley, C. R. (Ed.). (1995). *Compassion fatigue: Coping with secondary traumatic stress disorder in those who treat the traumatized.* New York, NY: Routledge

Figley, C. R., & Kleber, R. J. (1995). Beyond the "victim": Secondary traumatic stress. In R. F. Kleber, C.R. Figley, & Berthold P. Gersons (Eds.), *Beyond trauma: Cultural and societal dynamics* (pp. 75–98). New York, NY: Springer.

Figley, C. R. (2002a). Compassion fatigue: Psychotherapists' chronic lack of self-care. *Journal of Clinical Psychology, 58*(11), 1433–1441.

Figley, C. R. (Ed.). (2002b). *Treating compassion fatigue.* New York, NY: Brunner-Routledge.

Figley, C. R. (2007). *The art and science of caring for others without forgetting self-care.* Retrieved from http://www.giftfromwithin.org/html/artscien.html

Flarity, K. (2011). Compassion fatigue. *ENA Connection, 35*(7), 10.

Flarity, K., Gentry, J. E., & Mesnikoff, N. (2013). The effectiveness of an educational program on preventing and treating compassion fatigue in emergency nurses. *Advanced Emergency Nursing Journal, 35*(3), 247–258. doi:10.1097/TME.0b013e 31829b726f

Gentry, J. E. (2002). Compassion fatigue: A crucible of transformation. *Journal of Trauma Practice, 1*(3–4), 37–61.

Gentry, J. E. (2012). *Compassion fatigue prevention & resiliency: Fitness for the frontline course manual.* Retrieved from http://shop.pesi.com/product/compassionfatigue preventionandresiliencyfitnessforthefrontline%287286%29

Gentry, J. E., Baranowsky, A., & Dunning, K. (2002). The accelerated recovery program for compassion fatigue. In C. R. Figley (Ed.), *Treating compassion fatigue* (pp.123–138). New York, NY: Brunner-Routledge.

Gillespie, G. L., Gates, D. M., & Succop, P. (2010). Psychometrics of the healthcare productivity survey. *Advanced Emergency Nursing Journal, 32*(3), 258–271.

Hrivnak, E. (2013). *Wounded: A legacy of operation Iraqi freedom.* North Charleston, SC: CreateSpace Independent Publishing Platform.

Hooper, C., Craig, J., Janvrin, D. R., Wetsel, M. A., & Reimels, E. (2010). Compassion satisfaction, burnout, and compassion fatigue among emergency nurses compared with nurses in other selected inpatient specialties. *Journal of Emergency Nursing, 36*(5),420–427. doi:10.1016/j.jen.2009.11.027

Huggard, P. (2003). Compassion fatigue: How much can I give? *Medical Education, 37*(2), 163–164.

Laposa, J. M., Alden, L. E., & Fullerton, L. M. (2003). Work stress and posttraumatic stress disorder in ED nurses/personnel. *Journal of Emergency Nursing, 29*(1), 23–28.

Naparastek, B. (2006). *Invisible heroes: Survivors of trauma and how they heal.* New York, NY: Bantam Dell.

Pearlman, L. A., & Saakvitne, K. W. (1995). *Trauma and the therapist: Countertransference and vicarious traumatization in psychotherapy with incest survivors.* New York, NY: W. W. Norton.

Phipps, L. (1988). Stress among doctors and nurses in the emergency department of a general hospital. *Canadian Medical Association Journal, 139*(5), 375–376.

Rizzolatti G., & Fabbri-Destro, M. (2010). Mirror neurons: From discovery to autism. *Experimental Brain Research, 200*(3–4), 223–237. doi:10.1007/s00221-009-2002-3

Roney, L. (2010). *Compassion satisfaction and compassion fatigue among emergency department registered nurses* (Master's thesis). Retrieved from Dissertations & Theses: The Sciences and Engineering Collection (AAT 1486171).

Schwam, K. (1998). The phenomenon of compassion fatigue in perioperative nursing. *Association of Perioperative Registered Nurses Journal, 68*(4), 642–645, 647–648.

Stamm, B. H. (2009). *The ProQOL (Professional Quality of Life Scale: Compassion satisfaction and compassion fatigue version 5).* Retrieved from http://www.proqol.org/uploads/ProQOL_5_English.pdf

Stamm, B. H. (2010). *The concise ProQOL manual* (2nd ed.). Retrieved from http://www.proqol.org/uploads/ProQOL_Concise_2ndEd_12-2010.pdf

Stewart, D. W. (2009). Casualties of war: Compassion fatigue and health care providers. *Medical Surgical Nursing, 18*(2), 91–94.

Strommer, A. J. (2011). *Compassion fatigue and compassion satisfaction in emergency nurses in Alaska* (Unpublished master's thesis). Ann Arbor: University of Michigan.

Van Dernoot Lipsky, L., & Burk, C. (2009). *Trauma stewardship: An everyday guide to caring for self while caring for others.* San Francisco, CA: Berrett-Koehler.

Vaugh, D. (2005). *Wounds of war touch nurses.* Retrieved from http://news.nurse.com/article/20050117/DC/501170305

7

Micro-Costing Analysis of a Freestanding Birth Center: Development of a Data Collection Tool

Linda Cole, Kathryn Osborne, and Xiao Xu

DNP Essential #4

Information systems/technology and patient care technology for the improvement and transformation of health care

American Association of Colleges of Nursing. (2006). *The essentials of doctoral education for advanced nursing practice.* Retrieved from http://www.aacn.nche.edu/publications/position/DNPEssentials.pdf

This chapter describes the development of a data collection tool for microcosting provision of care within the freestanding birth center (FBC) model of maternity care.

It exemplifies DNP *Essential #4* as it relates to the use of information systems in improving health care.

Barbara A. Anderson, Editor

CAPSTONE FOCUS

The freestanding birth center (FBC) is an innovative model of care for low-risk childbearing women seeking minimal intervention outside the hospital setting. It is a small-business model that controls costs with short in-patient stays and minimal use of medical technology for low-risk patients. However, there have been few cost analyses, and no microcosting analysis, conducted on this maternity care model. This capstone focused on the development of a data collection tool for microcosting the FBC.

REVIEW OF THE LITERATURE

In the vast majority of cases, pregnancy and birth are healthy states. The birth center model promotes the wellness model of pregnancy within a home-like environment (American Association of Birth Centers [AABC], 2010). Studies on FBCs have demonstrated safety and excellent clinical outcomes (Brocklehurst et al., 2011; Rooks et al., 1989; Stapleton, Osborne & Illuzzi, 2013).

Consumer Demand for Birth Center Care

In the 1970s, modern FBCs opened in response to consumer desire for an alternative to the hospital for normal, physiologic birth. Most FBCs are state licensed and many are nationally accredited. Across the United States, birth centers are staffed with a variety of providers, including physicians, certified nurse-midwives (CNMs), and certified professional midwives (CPMs). Birth centers have grown in number from 195 in 2010 to 248 in 2013, which represents a 27% increase in 3 years (AABC. 2010). According to the National Center for Vital Statistics, between 2007 and 2010 the annual number of birth center births grew by 21.7%, during a time when overall births in the United States decreased by 7.3%. Though the popularity of this model of care is growing, the percentage of women who give birth in a birth center is extremely small (0.3% of the total births in the United States in 2010; United States Department of Health and Human Services, Centers for Disease Control and Prevention & National Center for Health Statistics, 2013).

Escalating Costs of Medical Care

Childbirth is the leading cause of hospitalization within the U.S. health care system, with mothers and newborns accounting for 23% of all hospital discharges. Six of the 15 most commonly performed procedures are associated with childbirth, and cesarean section is the most common in-patient surgical procedure performed. There are 4.3 million births annually in the United States and the cost of this care to society is immense (Sakala & Corry, 2008).

There is ongoing concern about the escalating costs of medical care in the United States. The inefficiency of the health care system impacts both cost of care and the overall health of the nation. It is vitally important to identify health care models that demonstrate both cost efficiency and quality outcomes. FBCs can meet both of these goals. Findings in the National Birth Center Study Part II showed decreases in both direct and indirect costs of care for maternity care (Rooks, Weatherby, & Ernst, 1992). Costs in birth centers are typically kept low by adhering to:

- A model of low-technology care
- Staffing managed in response to the ebb and flow of birth volume
- Early home discharge of mother and her baby

Birth Center Costs

Anderson and Anderson (1999) compared the costs of care in home, birth center, and hospital settings. The billable charges were used as a proxy for cost. Other studies also examined cost of birth center care only based upon billable charges, not actual costs (Frick, 2009; Scupholme & Kamons, 1987; Stone & Walker, 1995). This method of analysis measures what a birth center bills for care, which may be quite different from the actual cost of care. Other studies retrospectively examined data from accounting departments within birth centers, dividing fixed and variable costs and assigning a per-hour cost of care (Stone & Walker, 1997; Stone, Zwanziger, Hinton, Walker, & Buenting, 2000). This method lacks accuracy in measuring actual inputs into individual patient care.

The Centers for Medicare and Medicaid Services (CMS; 2013) has not clearly defined reimbursement for birth center facility or service charges, so there is no current Medicare- or Medicaid-derived reimbursement rate upon which to derive gross-costing figures. In addition, there is not an established cost estimate or fee schedule for birth center care. The conventional gross-costing approach for inpatient facilities is not practical in measuring costs in birth center care. Given that nearly half of all births in the United States (42.9%) are currently funded by Medicaid or the Children's Health Insurance Program (CHIP), it is worth considering the potential savings if more pregnant women receiving government-supported care gave birth in birth centers (CMS, 2013; Sakala & Corry, 2008).

Microcosting

Microcosting is a detailed method of collecting data that calls for the "direct enumeration and costing out of every input consumed in the treatment of a particular patient" (Weinstein, Siegel, Gold, Kamlet, & Russell, 1996, p. 188). Microcosting is considered the most accurate method of performing an economic analysis (Sarowar et al., 2010). "In principle, micro-costing (activity based costing or the bottom-up approach) is the preferred resource use measurement approach, in part because it is more reliable, accurate and flexible than more macro approaches" (Mogyorosy & Smith, 2005, p. 2).

The economic evaluation of health care is based on welfare economics, which is concerned with the impact of new services or models on the total welfare of society (Mogyorosy & Smith, 2005). Economic evaluations performed from a social perspective may include some additional cost items (e.g., patient productivity loss) that are not reflected in traditional accounting reports. In addition to medical costs, this societal perspective in cost analysis takes into consideration such costs incurred by the patient as travel time and expenses, patient out-of-pocket medication purchases, child care, time spent waiting for and receiving treatment, and decreased productivity or time away from work for the patient and/or family members (Smaldone, Tsimicalis, & Stone, 2011).

Microcosting is by nature a bottom-up approach rather than the traditional top-down approach of cost accounting. "Micro-costing data at the individual level are relevant for describing the precision of results in cost-effectiveness studies" (Frick, 2009, p. S77). Microcosting of FBCs could lead to comparative cost-and-effectiveness analyses of birth centers and hospitals. The essential elements of the microcosting approach are the collection of quantity and unit-cost data. The total cost of any given supply or service item comprising care is then estimated by multiplying the unit cost of the item by the total number of units consumed.

THE CAPSTONE PROJECT

The American Association of Birth Centers Foundation identified costing of birth center care as one of its funding priorities (Eunice [Kitty] Ernst, AABCF Board Member and founder of AABC, personal communication, January 2013). Eunice (Kitty) Ernst has purported:

> Health care reform is all about cost. The high quality care that birth centers provide is time-intensive care. The potential cost-benefit for investing in such care in the childbearing year, the beginning of life's journey, in terms of both immediate and long term benefits to the health and welfare of infants, mothers and families, and the health care system in general, are extraordinary and need to be analyzed. We must demonstrate our cost-savings. Someone has got to do a cost analysis of the birth center model! (personal communication, October 14, 2011)

The need for cost analysis fits with national health care priorities as well. The Institute of Medicine (IOM) included the freestanding birth center in the second quartile of *100 Initial Priority Topics for Comparative Effectiveness Research*. The need, as outlined by the IOM, is to compare the effectiveness of care in FBCs and the usual care of childbearing women at low and moderate risk (IOM, 2009). On February 15, 2013, the CMS awarded the AABC a $5.35 million, 4-year grant for the Strong Start for Mothers and Newborns Initiative, a funding opportunity to test the effectiveness of specific enhanced prenatal care approaches to reduce the frequency of premature births among pregnant Medicaid or CHIP beneficiaries at high risk for preterm births (CMS, 2013).

The timing of this DNP capstone project coincided well with the national initiative and the goals of AABC. At the time of the capstone project, the first author (LC) was serving as President of the American Association of Birth Centers and was also a DNP student. She was also practicing full-scope midwifery at the Lisa Ross Birth and Women's Center, Knoxville, Tennessee, a freestanding birth center operating for over 2 decades.

Goal of the Capstone Project

The Lisa Ross Birth and Women's Center has multiple programs tailored to the individual needs of clients, beginning with the first prenatal visit and ending with the 6-week postpartum visit for women. These programs include:

- Case management
- Group prenatal care

- Tailored length of visits
- Labor support, newborn care
- Home visits
- Breastfeeding support

The complexity of these resources at this FBC requires significant attention to detail. The goal of this DNP project was to develop a data collection tool for use in microcosting analysis at this FBC; the tool needed to capture both medical care and client costs.

Capstone Design

Cost items can be categorized as fixed or variable costs. Fixed costs are relatively independent of the volume of patients. Examples include salaried employees, space, utilities, marketing and outreach, licensure and accreditation, and contracted services such as accounting and grounds maintenance. Variable costs are expenses that change in proportion to the activity of a business. The more clients served, the more variable costs will be incurred. Using a societal approach applied to the FBC involves costing all aspects of the operations of the birth center. To facilitate a microcosting analysis from a societal perspective, the data collection tool needs to include both the costs of providing the service and the costs incurred by the client and her support system. Client-incurred costs could include, for example, time lost from work, transportation, child care, and doula services.

For the purpose of this tool development, cost data were generated from the following sources:

- The general ledger
- Accounting records
- Invoices
- Vendor supply lists

In order to approach the tool development from a societal perspective, three focus groups were conducted with women who received their prenatal care and delivered at the birth center in the preceding 6 months. A total of 17 women participated in the focus groups.

The Team

The development of this capstone project required the collaboration of a team of experts. The DNP capstone chair was Dr. Kathryn Osborne, professor at Frontier Nursing University. Dr. Osborne has served on the Board of Directors for the American College of Nurse Midwives and is widely published in the field of nurse–midwifery. Dr. Xiao Xu served as the content expert on the DNP capstone. Dr. Xu is an assistant professor in the Comparative Effectiveness Research Section of the Department of Obstetrics, Gynecology and Reproductive Sciences, Yale University. As a health economist and health services researcher, Dr. Xu's research focuses on improving the efficiency and outcomes of care for women and older adults. Her research projects have examined regional and hospital variations in cost of care; cost effectiveness of surgical, pharmacological, and behavioral interventions in women's health care; impact of insurance and other socioeconomic factors on health care utilization; health trajectories in older adults; and the influence of state medical liability environment on physicians' clinical practice. Dr. Xu's research has been funded by the Agency for Healthcare Research and Quality (AHRQ) and the Blue Cross Blue Shield of Michigan Foundation Collaboration with this capstone. Working with these experts exemplifies the benefit of networking and interdisciplinary collaboration.

After the initial proposal draft with committee chair, Dr. Osborne, LC spent 3 weeks at Yale University working closely with Dr. Xu on further refinement of the capstone project. Discussing key concepts of health economics and cost analysis with content expert, Dr. Xu, provided a rich immersion that added depth to the doctoral program.

Outcome

The full data collection tool was developed using microcosting of both operational and client costs. Its applicability was limited to the Lisa Ross Birth and Women's Center. In June 2013, LC was granted funding by AABC to conduct a pilot study of this data collection tool to measure birth center costs at the Lisa Ross Birth and Women's Center. The pilot study is in process. This project is a building block to accurate measurement of costs of the FBC model.

IMPACT

The data collection tool developed in this capstone project can be replicated and has potential in demonstrating the FBC as a cost-effective model of care. Findings from this study and subsequent analyses will help inform funders and legislators about the FBC as an innovative model of care, and a part of the solution for high-quality, high-value, client-centered care for low-risk pregnant women.

REFERENCES

American Association of Birth Centers. (2010). *Definition of a birth center* (Adopted October 1, 1995). Retrieved from http://www.birthcenters.org/about-aabc/posi tion-statements/definition-of-birth-center

Anderson, R. E., & Anderson, D. A. (1999). The cost-effectiveness of homebirth. *Journal of Nurse–Midwifery, 44*(1), 30–35.

Brocklehurst, P., Hardy, P., Hollowell, J., Linsell, L., Macfarlane, A., McCourt, C., . . . Stewart, M. [Birthplace in England Collaborative Group]. (2011). Perinatal and maternal outcomes by planned place of birth for healthy women with low risk pregnancies: The Birthplace in England national prospective cohort study. *British Medical Journal, 343*, d7400. doi:10.1136/bmj.d7400

Centers for Medicare and Medicaid Services. (2013). *Strong Start for Mothers and Newborns Initiative: Enhanced prenatal care models.* Retrieved from http://innovation. cms.gov/initiatives/Strong-Start-Strategy-2/index.html

Frick, K. D. (2009). Micro-costing quantity data collection methods. *Medical Care, 47*(7, Suppl. 1), S76–S81.

Institute of Medicine. (2009). *100 initial priority topics for comparative effectiveness research.* Retrieved from http://www.iom.edu/~/media/Files/Report%20Files/2009/ComparativeEffectivenessResearchPriorities/Stand%20Alone%20List%20of%20100%20CER%20Priorities%20-%20for%20web.ashx

Mogyorosy, Z., & Smith, P. (2005). *The main methodological issues in costing health care services: A literature review* (Centre for Heath Economics [CHE] Research Paper 7). York, England: University of York. Retrieved from http://www.york.ac.uk/che/pdf/rp7.pdf

Rooks, J. P., Weatherby, N. L., Ernst, E. K., Stapleton, S., Rosen, D., & Rosenfield, A. (1989). Outcomes of care in birth centers: The national birth center study. *New England Journal of Medicine, 321*(26), 1804–1811.

Rooks, J. P., Weatherby, N. L., & Ernst, E. K. (1992). National birth center study. Part II—Intrapartum and immediate postpartum and neonatal care. *Journal of Nurse–Midwifery, 37*(5), 301–330.

Sakala, C., & Corry, M. (2008). *Evidence-based maternity care: What it is and what it can achieve.* New York, NY: Childbirth Connection, the Reforming States Group, and the Milbank Memorial Fund. Retrieved from http://www.milbank.org/uploads/documents/0809MaternityCare/0809MaternityCare.html

Sarowar, M. G., Medin, E., Gazi, R., Koehlmoos, T. P., Rehnberg, C., Saifi, R., . . . Kahn, J. (2010). Calculation of costs of pregnancy- and puerperium-related care: Experience from a hospital in a low-income country. *Journal of Health, Population, and Nutrition, 28*(3), 264–272.

Smaldone, A., Tsimicalis, A., & Stone, P. W. (2011). Measuring resource utilization in patient-oriented comparative effectiveness research: A psychometric study of the resource utilization questionnaire. *Research and Theory for Nursing Practice: An International Journal, 25*, 80–106.

Scupholme, A., & Kamons, S. (1987). Are outcomes compromised when mothers are assigned to birth centers for care? *Journal of Nurse–Midwifery, 32*(4), 211–215.

Stapleton, S. R., Osborne, C., & Illuzzi, J. (2013). Outcome of care in birth centers: Demonstration of a durable model. *Journal of Midwifery & Women's Health, 58*(1), 3–14. doi:10.1111/jmwh.12003

Stone, P. W., & Walker, P. H. (1995). Cost-effectiveness analysis: Birth center vs. hospital care. *Nursing Economics, 13*(5), 299–308.

Stone, P. W., & Walker, P. H. (1997). Clinical and cost outcomes of a free-standing birth center: A comparison study. *Clinical Excellence for Nurse Practitioners, 1*(7), 456–465.

Stone, P. W., Zwanziger, J., Hinton Walker, P., & Buenting, J. (2000). Economic analysis of two models of low-risk maternity care: A freestanding birth center compared to traditional care. *Research in Nursing & Health, 23*(4), 279–289.

United States Department of Health and Human Services, Centers for Disease Control and Prevention & National Center for Health Statistics. (2013). *National vital statistics information.* Retrieved from http://www.cdc.gov/nchs/births.htm

Weinstein, M. C., Siegel, J., Gold, M. R., Kamlet, M. S., & Russell, L. B. (1996). Recommendations of the panel on cost-effectiveness in health and medicine. *The Journal of the American Medical Association, 276*, 1253–1258.

8

High-Fidelity Simulation in Graduate Education: Impact on Learning and Practice

Tia P. Andrighetti and Joyce M. Knestrick

DNP Essential #4

*Information systems/technology and patient care technology
for the improvement and transformation of health care*

American Association of Colleges of Nursing. (2006). *The essentials of doctoral education for advanced nursing practice.* Retrieved from http://www.aacn.nche.edu/publications/position/DNPEssentials.pdf

This chapter describes the development of an educational program using high-fidelity simulation for developing critical thinking skills among graduate nursing students and the subsequent expansion of this program into clinical practice.

It exemplifies DNP *Essential #4* as it relates to using information systems and technology to transform the learning environment in graduate education and clinical practice.

Joyce M. Knestrick, Editor

CAPSTONE FOCUS

Critical thinking, problem solving, and application of knowledge are essential to providing care for patients. The use of this skillset has a direct impact on the care provided by nurses. Various teaching methods are available to help teach nurses to think critically. One teaching method is the use of high-fidelity simulation.

Simulation is a methodology that is in widespread use in a variety of disciplines, including nursing and medicine. Early studies on simulation examined the use of simulation in the aviation industry to prepare for major untoward events experienced during flight. Later, medicine determined that if students were able to practice using simulated patients prior to real patient contact, less harm could occur to the patient. Simulations benefit the process of critical thinking, the application of knowledge, and the practice of clinical skills in a safe, nonthreatening environment (Berragan, 2011; Horan, 2009; Ravert, 2008). This capstone project focused on the use of high-fidelity simulation in both graduate education and in clinical practice to prepare nurses in optimal functioning and management of emergencies during birth.

REVIEW OF THE LITERATURE

Nurses apply knowledge, solve problems, and make critical decisions regarding patient care, often in an autonomous fashion. Since emergencies in childbirth do not necessarily present the same in all mothers, preparation in reacting to variations in presentation is essential. Rapid technological advances and emerging knowledge of abnormal birth processes necessitate that nurses possess critical thinking skills in adapting to new information (Institute of Medicine [IOM], 2010; Rash, 2008). The professional nurse, particularly the advanced practice registered nurse, must be able to critically appraise an emergent situation and gather resources to care for clients competently (Martin, 2002).

The use of simulation in the education of nurses is not new. Simple simulation techniques, such as learning to administer an injection into an orange, allowed nursing students to practice skills prior to patient contact. The advancement of technologically sophisticated simulations has not changed this basic premise, but the venues and tools have changed. There is a growing body of evidence on high-technology simulation (Brannan, White, & Bezanson, 2008; Horan, 2009; Ravert, 2008). There is, however, limited research on the use of high-technology simulation in the education of APNs, and outcome data exploring the use of high-fidelity simulation among health care providers is limited (Cook et al., 2011).

The National League for Nursing (NLN) and Laerdal Medical Company conducted a major nursing simulation study (Jeffries & Rizzolo, 2006). The purposes of this study were to identify nursing faculty who were using simulation, develop and test models to use during simulations, and contribute to the general body of knowledge on simulation technology. This study showed no significant increase in knowledge between students who learned with a static mannequin versus those with a high-fidelity mannequin. Student satisfaction was higher in the high-fidelity group. All students experiencing simulation learning had higher levels of confidence, and student-rated performance did not differ based on modality. The authors noted that ". . . active involvement and the opportunity to apply observational, assessment, and problem-solving skills, followed by a reflective thinking experience, leads to increased self-confidence in students" (Jeffries & Rizzolo, 2006, p. 12).

The National Council of State Boards of Nursing (NCSBN; 2013) is currently conducting a national multisite longitudinal study of simulation use in prelicensure nursing programs. This study is being done in three phases, with phase three currently undergoing implementation. The first phase involved surveying nursing programs to assess the percentage of time spent in simulations. The second phase of the study involved random assignment of students to one of three groups with varying amounts of simulation experience time. The first group engaged in clinical as usual, described as less than 10% of their time in simulations. The second group spent 25% of their clinical time in simulations, and the third group spent 50% of their time in simulations. Phase three follows the students after graduation into their first year of practice (NCSBN, 2013).

The results of this multisite study may determine the level of simulation used in nursing education programs. With increasing difficulty in obtaining clinical placements, especially in specialty areas, nursing students may spend 50% of their clinical time learning via the use of simulations. Prelicensure educators must become competent in incorporating simulation as a teaching methodology. Faculty who teach APNs will also be affected, as the nurses attending graduate school may be accustomed to using simulation methods and have expectations of simulation in graduate education.

A core competency for nurse educators, according to the NLN (2006), is the ability to ". . . create opportunities for learners to develop their critical thinking and critical reasoning skills" (p. 1). Modalities to develop these skills have dominated the nursing education literature. The American Association of Colleges of Nursing (AACN) 2008 policy statement for baccalaureate nurses mentions critical thinking as a needed element in educating nurses and identifies simulation as a critical thinking modality. If these skills are essential at the baccalaureate level, then higher levels of critical thinking and reasoning skills are necessary at the graduate level, especially when preparing APNs for autonomous roles. In order to meet these competencies, nursing education programs at all levels are utilizing simulation modalities.

The Institute of Medicine (IOM) report, *The Future of Nursing: Leading Change, Advancing Health* (2010), is a blueprint for national transformation to ensure appropriate health care (2010). This groundbreaking report calls for many changes, including nursing education focused on interdisciplinary teamwork competencies and the advancement of critical thinking skills for the management of complex patient situations. The report calls for nursing education programs to prepare nurses to practice to the full extent of their education, guiding patients in the prevention and management of disease. This is a daunting task for currently understaffed nursing education programs across the nation. The IOM supports the use of simulation as one method to facilitate this educational transformation (IOM, 2010).

High-Fidelity Simulation

Since nursing students at all levels are expected to spend much of their clinical time in simulation activities, educators need to make simulation experiences as close to actual clinical situations as possible. There is a distinction between a *high-fidelity simulator* and a *high-fidelity simulation*. A high-fidelity simulator is a mannequin with life-like qualities. A high-fidelity simulation is a scenario with life-like reenactment (Beaubien & Baker, 2004). It uses the environment and props to simulate a life-like scenario that encourages participants to suspend reality and enter into the simulated experience (Berragan, 2011; Lathrop, Winningham, & VandeVusse, 2007). It facilitates practice with communication and teamwork (Berragan, 2011).

According to Beaubien and Baker (2004), high-fidelity simulation promotes the development of skills needed to handle complex clinical and emergent situations.

By first practicing skills in a safe, nonthreatening environment, the student is able to apply the skills and information gained in the classroom setting. The student is then given feedback about skills and interaction with patients and family as well as team leadership. There is a growing realization that simulation is a valuable experience for students who may not encounter rare complications during clinical rotations and only occasionally in future practice (Hyland, Weeks, Ficorelli, &, Vandermeek-Warren, 2012). Simulations also enable nursing educators to provide the practice opportunities where no harm can be done, while students are waiting for appropriate learning situations in clinical sites. Since clinical placements are becoming increasingly harder to find, this method of clinical skill acquisition is becoming essential (Hyland et al., 2012; Miller & Bull, 2013).

Stress in the clinical setting can deeply affect students. A benefit of high-fidelity simulation is that it can create the stress of a crisis by reenacting an actual clinical crisis (Lathrop et al., 2007; Norris, 2008). The ability to reenact this stress not only gives the student a realistic idea of the emotional impact of the stress, but also equips the student to deal with that stress. Repetition and practice in a safe, nonthreatening environment helps to ameliorate these stressful feelings (Lathrop et al., 2007).

The effects of stress during flight were originally studied by the aviation industry. Using a high-fidelity simulation experience, it was discovered that aviation students learned better if stress began in a low-pressure environment and escalated over time (Keinan, Friedland, & Sarig-Naor, 1990). Extrapolating this learning to the health care environment, the student starts with readings on a topic, moves to a discussion of those readings and demonstration of management, and then participates in a high-fidelity simulation with gradual escalation in stress. This method accommodates a variety of learning styles, allows time for learning, and enhances muscle memory.

Benefits of High-Fidelity Simulation in Clinical Setting Skills Acquisition

The use of simulation is a beneficial method in skill acquisition prior to an actual client encounter (Berragan, 2011; Horan, 2009; Ravert, 2008) or in preparing for clinical situations that occur infrequently (Brannan et al., 2008; Horan, 2009). Simulation also allows for skill acquisition prior to actual patient contact in a situation where potential harm is a significant factor (Horan, 2009; Miller & Bull, 2013; Ravert, 2008). This skill acquisition is especially important with high-stakes skills, such as surgery, obstetrics, catheterizations, and medication administration. Simulations may help practitioners diagnose a complication earlier, make an appropriate assessment of the situation, and gather needed resources in a more timely manner while practicing communication with other members of the health care team. A meta-analysis examining technology-enhanced simulation use in the education of health professionals compared to no intervention found moderate to large statistically significant positive results of technology-enhanced simulation on clinician behaviors and patient care outcomes (Cook et al., 2011).

Interprofessional Education

The World Health Organization (WHO, 2010) defines interprofessional education (IPE) as follows: ". . . when students from two or more professions learn about, from and with each other to enable effective collaboration and improve health outcomes" (p. 7). WHO states that educating practitioners in working together during their education period will enable smoother communication and more collaborative practice after graduation. It has set a goal of having ". . . collaborative, practice-ready health care workers" (WHO, 2010, p. 7). By having practice-ready new graduates who are well-versed in working with other health care team members, the transition from school to work environment is facilitated.

Interprofessional learning needs to occur, not only with students, but also with practicing health professionals, especially those caring for patients who require skills delivered through teamwork. As an educational approach, IPE helps each team member to understand the role and scope of practice of the other team members. Credentialing bodies (Accreditation Commission for Education in Nursing [ACEN], 2013; AACN, 2011) frequently require this approach. The Joint Commission on Accreditation of Healthcare Organizations (JCAHO) has noted lack of communication as a remediation issue following untoward events (JCAHO, 2004). Simulation may promote greater patient safety, addressing the clarion call by the IOM to reduce medical errors (Kohn, Corrigan, & Donaldson, 1999).

Competency Assessment

Employing institutions can benefit from the use of simulation in the orientation of newly hired nurses. The profession of nursing is also looking for a way to assess competency of practicing nurses. In 2005 the NCSBN called for reform of the current process, with simulation as a way to assess that competency (Decker, 2011). Simulation can document competencies and allow the employer to individualize orientation. It could also potentially shorten orientation time and allow for quicker entry into practice. Simulation has also been used in the interview process and as a structured assessment tool for advancement as a way of determining skills and competencies (Mitchell, Strube, Vaux, West, & Auditore, 2013). Many specialty organizations currently use simulation to determine ongoing competency assessment (American Heart Association, 2013; Neonatal Resuscitation Program, 2012).

THE CAPSTONE PROJECT

As nursing educators, both authors have worked with students prior to clinical immersion. We have observed a need to enhance skill development and make it as lifelike as possible through both hands-on practice and simulations. Such practice enables the student to not only practice skills, but also to learn about management of unpredictable situations.

Overview of the Capstone Project

As part of her DNP capstone project, the first author (TA) explored the use of high-fidelity simulations in increasing nurse–midwifery students' confidence in the management of obstetrical complications, specifically shoulder dystocia and postpartum hemorrhage (PPH) management. These complications can be sudden and life-threatening, with no anticipated risk factors (Cunningham et al., 2010). Therefore, graduate students studying nurse–midwifery must be taught how to handle these emergencies. The project was conducted at Frontier Nursing University (FNU), a community-based, distance learning graduate program. The University builds all curricula upon the Community of Inquiry Model, a model of active learning (see Garrison, Anderson, & Archer, 1999). The University was supportive of this simulation project to promote active learning.

Study Design

A preliminary needs assessment revealed that a significant portion of nurse-midwifery students at the University were graduating with no clinical experience in managing either PPH or shoulder dystocia. Even if these events did occur in the process of clinical exposure, the literature identifies that, across the nation, preceptors appropriately step in and assume care of at-risk mothers in order to ensure an optimal outcome (Lathrop et al., 2007). However, without some experience with managing these life-threatening events, students, upon graduation, may be forced to handle these complications for the first time on their own.

Project Goals

Four capstone project goals were identified:

- To provide opportunities for nurse–midwifery students at FNU to apply knowledge about shoulder dystocia and PPH management
- To ensure practice of these two complications prior to an actual high-stakes encounter
- To assess the impact of high-fidelity simulation on the development of student confidence in the management of shoulder dystocia and PPH
- To contribute to the body of knowledge on high-fidelity simulation use in nurse–midwifery education

Theoretical Model

Simulation can be a powerful tool in helping adult learners visualize concepts and apply knowledge in a safe, nonthreatening environment prior to facing an actual crisis in the care of a birthing woman. The conceptual framework selected for the project was Knowles Adult Learning Theory, which specifically describes approaches to help adult learners visualize the interconnectedness of concepts and applications of knowledge to actual life situations (Knowles & Associates, 1984). Simulation scenarios for management of PPH and shoulder dystocia were developed using adult learning theory, best practices for simulation, and evidence-based management of obstetric complications. Scripts were written to promote standardization of simulation activities. A comprehensive equipment list was developed and a simulation teaching room was equipped.

Evaluation Tool

The study conducted by the National League for Nursing (NLN) and Laerdal Medical Company (Jeffries & Rizzolo, 2006) produced many tested tools for use with simulations including the Student Satisfaction and Self-Confidence in Learning tool. These tools have content validity and reliability. The Student Satisfaction and Self-Confidence in Learning tool was not designed as an obstetrical pre-/posttest tool. Permission was obtained from the NLN to adapt the tool to accommodate use in nurse–midwifery education and to adjust the pre-/posttest format.

Implementation

During the project, one of the two authors attended three 4-day, on-campus clinical education sessions in order to gather data and to implement the project. In the first session, the first author collected baseline data on student confidence levels in the management of shoulder dystocia and PPH as 10 students in the control group engaged in the usual traditional simulations. In the second and third sessions, the first author implemented the third goal using the scripted scenarios with 18 students in the high-fidelity intervention group. Student confidence levels were compared with this intervention in contrast to the usual or high-fidelity educational intervention.

Project Outcome

The first goal of this capstone project was to provide opportunities for nurse-midwifery students to apply knowledge about shoulder dystocia and PPH management. This goal was met in both groups by student–faculty discussion, faculty demonstration of management, and student participation in simulation. The second goal was timing the practice of these two complications prior to an actual high-stakes encounter. Again, this goal was accomplished with every student. Additional practice time was built into the simulation for students who did not receive the scenario where major maneuvers were involved. The third goal was to assess the impact of high-fidelity simulation on the development of student confidence in the management of shoulder dystocia and PPH. This study's findings showed the following:

There was a small increase in the confidence scores between the pretest and posttest for the control group, but the increase was not statistically significant for either the shoulder dystocia or PPH simulations. In contrast, posttest scores were significantly ($P < .01$) higher for the intervention group. When the pretest and posttest change scores were compared for the control and intervention groups, there was a moderate effect size (0.54) in the intervention group for the shoulder dystocia simulations and a large effect size (1.68) for the PPH simulations (Andrighetti, Knestrick, Marowitz, Martin, & Engstrom, 2012, p. 57).

The results of this project indicate that student confidence is enhanced with the use of high-fidelity simulations. While high-fidelity simulation, at this point, has not been shown to necessarily equate to safer outcomes for patients, it is a step needed to decrease immobilizing fear in an emergent situation. Students reported feeling afraid during the simulations and described how completing the simulations helped them to work through their fears.

The fourth goal of the project was to contribute to the body of knowledge on high-fidelity simulation use in nurse–midwifery education. This capstone project was published in the *Journal of Midwifery and Women's Health* (Andrighetti et al., 2012). This capstone project exemplifies DNP *Essential #4* as it relates to using information systems and technology to transform the learning environment in graduate education and clinical practice.

PROJECT EXPANSION TO THE CLINICAL SETTING

As part of the practicum component of the doctoral program, the first author worked with a local hospital in Concord, New Hampshire. I approached the obstetrical (OB) nurse educator about the possibility of implementing obstetrical high-fidelity simulations among the nursing staff. This discussion coincided with the hospital opening a simulation lab. As none of the simulation educators had obstetrical experience, I offered to fill that role. As a nurse–midwife highly experienced in maternity care, a nursing educator, and now completing my DNP capstone work on high-fidelity simulation with obstetrical emergencies, I felt qualified.

The family practice attending physician from Dartmouth University heard about my project and approached the OB nurse educator, asking if the family practice residents could participate. I modified the scripts for the student-based simulation on shoulder dystocia and PPH to fit with the experience levels of the labor and delivery nurses as well as the residents and began to run these interdisciplinary simulations. For instance, there was a scenario in which the resident was paged to a birthing room for a shoulder dystocia and the interdisciplinary team responded. Transferring this learning modality from the graduate nursing classroom to the hospital-based simulation center with practicing health professionals is an example of interdisciplinary simulations, using technology to bring together ". . . collaborative, practice-ready health care workers" (WHO, 2010, p. 7).

The simulation template was shared with Concord Hospital's simulation center and the family practice attending physician. I was able to observe providers I did not know reenacting my scenarios. I also noticed that during the debriefing, participants who had read my scenarios used the scenarios to discuss certain aspects such as closed-loop communication and the rationale for the debriefing exercise.

On the last day of my involvement at this site, the person who played the role of the patient during the simulation was not available, so I played the standardized patient role, acting as a women giving birth. Playing this role gave me an appreciation for the unforeseen impact that the educator can have on learners. During the simulation of shoulder dystocia, the family practice resident told me she was going to give me an episiotomy. I loudly told her that we had talked about that during my prenatal care and I did not want one. The visibly startled resident did not know what to do, but my reaction forced her to rethink the plan and explain her rationale for cutting the episiotomy. This experience gave her a simulated opportunity to communicate with a woman during a birth complication. By playing dual roles as birthing mother with a complication and simulation educator, the resident and I both experienced a teaching moment.

CONCLUSION

Experience in running simulations led both authors into deeper insight into the learning process. We learned that the critical factor in simulation education is thinking in the moment, keeping the simulations running, and responding to the unexpected. I also learned that the debriefing process is an art, guiding students and practicing health professionals in analysis of the simulated event.

Developing critical thinking skills is an art and a science. Using the technology of high-fidelity simulation has great potential for building these skills as well as assessing competency in the clinical setting. In order to accurately measure competency, scripts, equipment lists, and simulation procedures need to be standardized.

REFERENCES

Accreditation Commission for Education in Nursing. (2013). *Accreditation manual.* Retrieved from http://acenursing.org/accreditation manual

American Association of Colleges of Nursing. (2008). *The essentials of baccalaureate education for professional nursing practice.* Retrieved from www.aacn.nche.edu/Education/pdf/BaccEssentials08.pdf

American Association of Colleges of Nursing. (2011). *The essentials of master's education in nursing.* Retrieved from http://www.aacn.nche.edu/education-resources/MastersEssentials11.pdf

American Heart Association. (2013). *BLS for healthcare providers—Classroom.* Retrieved from http://www.heart.org/HEARTORG/CPRAndECC/HealthcareProviders/BasicLifeSupportBLS/BLS-for-Healthcare-Providers---Classroom_UCM_303484_Article.jsp

Andrighetti, T. P., Knestrick, J. M., Marowitz, A., Martin, C., & Engstrom, J. L. (2012). Shoulder dystocia and postpartum hemorrhage simulations: Student confidence in managing these complications. *Journal of Midwifery and Women's Health, 57*(1), 55–60. doi:10.1111/j.1542-2011.2011.00085.x.

Beaubien, J. M., & Baker, D. P. (2004). The use of simulation for training teamwork skills in health care: How low can you go? *Quality and Safety in Health Care, 13*(Suppl. 1), 151–156.

Berragan, L. (2011). Simulation: An effective pedagogical approach for nursing? *Nurse Education Today, 31*(7), 660–663. doi:10.1016/j.nedt.2011.01.019.

Brannan, J. D., White, A., & Bezanson, J. L. (2008). Simulator effects on cognitive skills and confidence levels. *Journal of Nursing Education, 47*(11), 495–500.

Cook, D. A., Hatala, R., Brydges, R., Zendejas, B., Szostek, J. H., Wang, A. T., . . . Hamstra, S. J. (2011). Technology-enhanced simulations for health professions education. *Journal of the American Medical Association, 306*(9), 978–988. doi:10. 1001/jama.2011.1234.

Cunningham, F. G., Leveno, K. J., Bloom, S. L., Hauth, J. C., Rouse, D. J., & Spong, C. Y. (2010). *Williams Obstetrics* (23rd ed.). New York, NY: McGraw-Hill.

Decker, S., Utterback, V. A., Thomas, M. B., Mitchell, M., & Sportsman, S. (2011). Assessing continued competency through simulation: A call for stringent action. *Nursing Education Perspectives, 32*(2), 120–125. doi:http://dx.doi.org/10.5480/ 1536-5026-32.2.120

Fahey, J. O., & Mighty, H. E. (2008). Shoulder dystocia: Using simulation to train providers and teams. *Journal of Perinatal & Neonatal Nursing, 22*(2), 114–122. doi:10.1097/01. JPN.0000319097.05415.1d

Garrison, D. R., Anderson, T., & Archer, W. (1999). Critical inquiry in a text-based environment: Computer conferencing in higher education. *The Internet and Higher Education, 2*(2–3), 87–105.

Horan, K. M. (2009). Using the human patient simulator to foster critical thinking in critical situations. *Nursing Education Perspectives, 30*(1), 28–30.

Hyland, D., Weeks, B. H., Ficorelli, C. T., & Vanderbeek-Warren, M. (2012). Bringing simulationto life. *Teaching and Learning in Nursing, 7*(3), 108–112.

Institute of Medicine. (2010). *The future of nursing: Leading change, advancing health.* Washington, DC: National Academies Press. Retrieved from http://www.iom .edu/Reports/2010/The-future-of-nursing-leading-change-advancing-health .aspx

Jeffries, P. R., & Rizzolo, M. A. (2006). *Summary report: Designing and implementing models for the innovative use of simulation to teach nursing care of ill adults and children: A national, multi-site, multi-method study.* Retrieved from http://www.nln.org/ researchgrants/LaerdalReport.pdf

Joint Commission on Accreditation of Healthcare Organizations. (2004). Sentinel event alert Issue 30: Preventing infant death and injury during delivery. Retrieved from http://www.jointcommission.org/assets/1/18/SEA_30.PDF

Keinan, G., Friedland, N., & Sarig-Naor, V. (1990). Training for task performance under stress: The effectiveness of phase training methods. *Journal of Applied Social Psychology, 20*(18), 1514–1529. doi:10.1111/j.1559-1816.1990.tb01490.x

Knowles, M. S., & Associates. (1984). *Andragogy in action: Applying modern principles of adult learning theory.* San Francisco, CA: Jossey-Bass.

Kohn, L. T., Corrigan, J. M., &. Donaldson, M. S. (Eds.). (2000). *To err is human: Building a safer health system.* Washington, DC: The National Academies Press. Retrieved from http://www.iom.edu/Reports/1999/to-err-is-human-building-a-safer-health-system.aspx

Lathrop, A., Winningham, B., & VandeVusse, L. (2007). Simulation-based learning for midwives: Background and pilot implementation. *Journal of Midwifery and Women's Health, 52*(5), 492–498.

Martin, C. (2002). The theory of critical thinking of nursing. *Nursing Education Perspectives, 23*(5), 243–247.

Miller, A., & Bull, R. M. (2013). Do you want to play? Factors influencing nurse academics' adoption of simulation in their teaching practices. *Nurse Education Today, 33*(3), 241–246. doi:10.1016/j.nedt.2011.11.001

Mitchell, M., Strube, P. M., Vaux, A. M., West, N. G., & Auditore, A. (2013). Right person, right skills, right job: The contribution of objective structured clinical examinations in advancing staff nurse experts. *Journal of Nursing Administration, 43*(10), 543–548. doi:10.1016/j.nedt.2011.11.001

National Council of State Boards of Nursing. (2013). *NCSBN national simulation study.* Retrieved from https://www.ncsbn.org/2094.htm

National League for Nursing. (2005). *Core competencies of nurse educators with task statements.* Retrieved from http://www.nln.org/profdev/corecompetencies.pdf

Neonatal Resuscitation Program. (2012). *Simulation.* Retrieved from http://www2.aap.org/NRP/simulation.html

Norris, G. (2008). The midwifery curriculum: Introducing obstetric emergency simulation. *British Journal of Midwifery, 16*(4), 232–235.

Rash, E. M. (2008). A problem based learning hybrid in a women's health course. *Journal of Nursing Education, 47*(10), 477–479.

Ravert, P. (2008). Patient simulator sessions and critical thinking. *Journal of Nursing Education, 47*(12), 557–562.

World Health Organization, Health Professions Networks Nursing and Midwifery Office. (2010). *Framework for action on interprofessional education and collaborative practice.* Retrieved from http://whqlibdoc.who.int/hq/2010/WHO_HRH_HPN_10.3_eng.pdf

9

Medicare Reimbursement and the Nurse Practitioner: An Issue of Equity

Gigi Whaley-Pryor

DNP Essential #5

Health care policy for advocacy in health care

American Association of Colleges of Nursing. (2006). *The essentials of doctoral edu-cation for advanced nursing practice.* Retrieved from http://www.aacn.nche.edu/publications/position/DNPEssentials.pdf

This chapter describes the development of educational materials targeting policy makers in the federal government on the limitations of "incident to" billing for nurse practitioner services.

It exemplifies DNP *Essential #5* as it relates to advocacy for just reimbursement for nurse practitioner practice.

Barbara A. Anderson, Editor

CAPSTONE FOCUS

This capstone focused on the need for education of policy makers on "inci-dent to" billing within the Medicare reimbursement system. Medicare billing for nurse practitioner (NP) services works in two different ways: *direct billing,* where the NP bills under an individual national provider identification (NPI) number, and *"incident to" billing.* In order to bill as an "incident to," a health care delivery service must be identified as a physician service in which a non-physician provides service (Gosfield, 2001). Medicare "incident to" rules were developed in order to cover provided services that are "an integral, although 'incident to,' part of the physician's professional services to the patient" (Gosfield, 2001, p. 24). "Incident to" billing is an unfair reimbursement practice that obstructs the provision of care by NPs who attend Medicare recipients. Further, it is a significant barrier to the promotion and advancement of advanced practice nursing.

REVIEW OF THE LITERATURE

The NP in the Health Care System

In the visionary report, *The Future of Nursing: Leading Change, Advancing Health*, the Institute of Medicine (IOM) calls for a greater leadership role of nurses in America's increasingly complex and changing health care system (IOM, 2011). The IOM (2011) report supports the evolution of policy to strengthen the practice of the NP as a crucial team member in improving and maintaining the health of all ages served by the American health care system (IOM, 2011). The report calls for the removal of practice laws that prohibit NPs from delivering care to the full extent of certification, education, and training. Further, it references the growing population, including Medicare recipients and the elderly, who continue to experience limited access to health care (IOM, 2011). Limited access is a growing concern within the field of primary care, specifically affecting certain underserved patient populations, including inner-city populations, rural areas, and elderly patients (Lee, 2011).

Since the 1977 Rural Health Clinic Services Act, NPs and physician's assistants (PAs) have served as providers, under physician supervision, meeting the needs of patients in a variety of settings. Soon after this Act, NP certification allowed NPs to maintain autonomous practice in which they could see patients independently of physician supervision, and NP practice sites expanded from rural settings to underserved urban areas (Weiland, 2008).

The Effectiveness of NP Care

Delgado-Passler and McCaffrey (2006) examined NP-directed telemanagement programs for heart failure patients compared to registered nurse-directed programs, demonstrating the potential benefits of NP care for Medicare patients. This study provided an introduction to NP management of heart failure patients and NP postdischarge management aiming to decrease hospital readmission. Specifically, the authors demonstrated that an NP-directed heart failure telemanagement program can reduce the rising costs of frequent admissions. The authors also reviewed previous studies demonstrating that NP postdischarge management is effective in reducing cost and readmissions. While one study reviewed did not demonstrate this effect, the authors determined that the study was not biased against NP care (Delgado-Passler & McCaffrey, 2006).

Mezey et al. (2005) found corroborating evidence of the benefits of NPs in the care of geriatric populations. This study reviewed a national survey of nursing home medical directors conducted by the John A. Hartford Foundation Institute for Geriatric Nursing (Hartford Institute). The Hartford Institute's survey described the efficacy of practice patterns of NPs in nursing homes in order to advocate for strengthening their use in such locations (Mezey et al., 2005).

Lee (2011) described the effectiveness of NP involvement in health care, stressing the centrality of NP autonomy without supervisory and collaborative clauses. "The effective use of NPs could help alleviate the current health care crisis by providing patients with access to excellent health care at reasonable rates" (Lee, 2011, p. 764). Through examination of federal and state laws governing the scope of nursing practice, Lee (2011) concluded, "The care provided to patients by NPs matches or exceeds the care provided by physicians in a variety of settings, such as retail clinics, minor emergency areas, and rural health clinics" (p. 766). This conclusion corroborates with the findings of Mezey et al. (2005). Lee (2011) suggested expansion of autonomous NP services into telemedicine, cybermedicine, telehealth, and telenursing. The author concluded, "To effectively provide care to individuals, NPs need the autonomy to deliver competent care independent from that of physicians" (Lee, 2011, p. 768).

Economic Efficiency and Medicare

Economic efficiency theory states that organizations should structure their output to achieve the lowest possible cost per unit produced (QFinance, 2013). Extrapolating to Medicare, services (the output) should be structured to provide the lowest costs per Medicare patient (the unit). Primary care and preventative services efficiently achieve lower costs (QFinance, 2013).

Efficient allocation of resources is essential. Economists define three types of efficient allocation of resources: *technical, allocative,* and *productive* (Zhang, Unruh, & Wan, 2008). Technical efficiency is defined as "the maximum possible output from a given set of inputs" (Zhang et al., 2008, p. 1045), that is, services provided to Medicare patients. Allocative efficiency is defined as "the most efficient combination of inputs given their prices and production technology" (Zhang et al., 2008, p. 1045). For Medicare, this would mean the costs of services provided by Medicare providers. Productive efficiency is defined as "when both technological and allocative efficiency exist" (Zhang et al., 2008, p. 1045). Within the Medicare system, productive efficiency requires an adequate supply of providers to meet the needs of Medicare patients. The author has noted that the current overuse of specialists and lack of primary care providers for Medicare patients results in higher costs.

Since the early 1990s, Medicare funding has been tied to a preset target. This target was based on the volume performance standard (a legal amount designated annually) and the sustainable growth rate (SGR; Wilensky, 2009). As the number of Medicare primary care physicians declines, there is an increasing mismatch (Weiland, 2008). NPs currently serve many patients in the growing Medicare pool. The utilization of NPs is essential in order to provide skilled and knowledgeable care to this growing population (Sullivan-Marx, 2008). NPs can provide an adequate workforce to meet the needs of Medicare patients (Jacobs, 1996). However, that will not occur unless the NPs receive adequate reimbursement.

Reimbursement for NP Services Within the Medicare System

Working within the current rules of Medicare, the reimbursement rate for the "incident to" method of billing for NPs is 100% if undersigned by a physician. However, if the NP bills Medicare under his or her NPI number, the NP is paid at a 15% lower rate than the physician for providing the same services and procedures (Frakes & Evans, 2006; Hull-Grommesh, Ellis, & Mackey, 2010). This Medicare reimbursement policy deters NPs from providing autonomous primary care to Medicare patients. The "incident to" billing method allows the physician to bill at 100%, enhancing his or her income and promoting billing at the maximal rate that does not benefit the patient or the cost-effectiveness of the health care system.

This cascade of events drives NPs toward attending to privately insured patients instead of Medicare-insured patients in order to increase their income and to offset the financial loss associated with Medicare reimbursement (Weiland, 2008). Further, current practice requires the Medicare patient to have two providers at once, one in a supervisory role and another in the care provider role. Having more than one provider involved for a Medicare service is confusing for many patients, is not cost effective, complicates billing, and produces widespread Medicare fraud (O'Grady & Brassard, 2011).

Studies of "Incident to" Billing

Gosfield (2001) reviewed "incident to" billing among physicians working with nonphysician providers. The review addressed the history, requirements, coding, and documentation of "incident to" billing. In addition, risk for Medicare fraud, direct billing by nonphysician providers, the cost of poor coding, and legal implications were reviewed. The author concluded that all personnel needed better understanding of the process (Gosfield, 2001).

Chapman, Wides, and Spetz (2010) reviewed the history of the Medicare payment system and Medicare reimbursement, including "incident to" reimbursement and independent billing by NPs. The authors concluded that a better payment system was necessary, maximizing the use of NPs and decreasing the risk of Medicare fraud. Edmunds (2002) also examined reimbursement disparity, demonstrating that with "incident to" billing, the physician receives a full fee without seeing the patient. The significance of "incident to" billing is that NPs are viewed as dependent practitioners, justifying lower rates. In turn, as NPs are employed by physicians, the NP work is not traceable, NPs do not have a voice, and the physician is credited for the work he or she does (Weiland, 2008).

Weiland (2008) examined factors influencing the ability of NPs to practice as independent primary care providers. The author examined authority and role issues between the physician and the NP within a historical context. The author identified existing disparity in Medicare reimbursement as key to independent practice, stating, "The outcome for reimbursement policy and current reimbursement practices is that 95% of NPs function within an employee role, and only 2% to 4% of NPs practice in an independently operated NP clinic" (Weiland, 2008, p. 350).

THE CAPSTONE PROJECT

Prior to learning about "incident to" billing in my DNP program at the University of Utah, I had limited interest in the billing process and I was unaware of this inequitable practice. The coursework in one class brought an epiphany. I felt angry with the message of lesser value ascribed to NPs within the Medicare system. I began to ask NPs about their views on "incident to" billing. A few NPs reported they refused to allow their services to be billed as "incident to" and worked completely autonomously, as the state of Utah allows. The majority, however, stated that this was the status quo and that they did not want to "rock the boat." Many worked in clinics owned or dominated by physicians or by hospital corporations that catered to physician satisfaction and maintenance of the status quo. My professors predicted that "incident to" billing would eventually be legislated out of practice, but most of them stated it would not happen within the timeframe of their careers.

The purpose of this capstone project was to advocate for just reimbursement for NPs serving Medicare patients. I focused on informing Congressional members about the inequity of "incident to" billing and its effect on the practice of NPs. This approach was in coherence with DNP *Essential #5, Health care policy for advocacy in health care* (American Association of Colleges of Nursing [AACN], 2006).

Not finding any existing white papers on this topic, I developed a white paper supported by a fact sheet. The fact sheet was a rapid way of disseminating information to members of Congress. The fact sheet became the most valuable tool in the project. The educational materials outlined the value of the NP in reducing costs while increasing the ranks of available health care providers for the Medicare population. The white paper called for a policy change providing equity in reimbursement as both an issue of social justice and as a means of ensuring an adequate pool of skilled providers.

I sent a letter of introduction, the white paper, and the fact sheet to targeted members of Congress via fax. Due to security risks, hard copies could not be mailed and the material could not be e-mailed, as only constituents within a congressman's district can e-mail their senator or representative. The only exception was the ability to send hard copies to Utah members of Congress, as this project was conducted at the University of Utah.

A total of 68 faxes were sent to 64 individual members of the Senate and House of Representatives and various Congressional groups responsible for Medicare policy. These groups included the U.S. Senate Finance committee; Health, Education, Labor and Pensions committee; Ways and Means committee; and the subcommittee on Commerce, Manufacturing, and Trade. By faxing to these committees, the materials reached all staff of Congress members responsible for Medicare policy change. The timeline for response was 2 months from the time of information dissemination.

The majority of Congress members did not acknowledge receipt of any communications. Of the total of seven responses from Congressmen, only two responded to the issue, that is, "incident to" billing.

IMPACT

The outcomes of this project demonstrated the barriers to communication in the current heath policy arena. Even though all members of Congress are responsible for voting on health care policy changes, a citizen can only readily contact his or her own senators and representatives. Due to the daily volume of communication, legislators only respond to constituents. This project demonstrated that, as a body, members of Congress cannot be contacted by individual citizens, such as NPs or Medicare recipients, who are affected by a change in legislation and policy.

The greatest lesson learned from this policy project was the need for professional grouping and lobbying in the process of advocating for policy change. NPs need to participate in professional organizations in order to lobby and advocate for equity in pay. The topics of equity in pay and autonomous practice will continue to surface as health care costs escalate among Medicare recipients. NPs are now uniting as one entity under the Consensus Model. This creates a uniform, organized voice moving the profession toward equity in pay and autonomous practice.

Coalition building is essential, especially with senior citizen groups. The AARP, the American Public Health Association (APHA), Utah Nurse Practitioners (UNP), and the American Academy of Nurse Practitioners (AANP) are advocacy groups that share a vision for Medicare reform. NPs need to work with all these organizations as one voice to change the status of "incident to" billing.

CONCLUSION

This DNP capstone project raised my awareness about the strength of professional associations working together for a shared vision. Currently, the Medicare health care system is very strained, in need of change in order to plan for and provide patient care (O'Brien, 2011). In order to strengthen advanced practice nursing and to broaden the scope of practice in individual states and nationally via Medicare reimbursement, NPs need to use their influence with law makers. By deleting the "incident to" billing approach and promoting autonomous practice among NPs, the growing numbers of Medicare recipients will be better served.

REFERENCES

American Association of Colleges of Nursing. (2006). *The essentials of doctoral education for advanced nursing practice.* Retrieved from http://www.aacn.nche.edu/publications/position/DNPEssentials.pdf

Chapman, S. A., Wides, C. D., & Spetz, J. (2010). Payment regulations for advanced practice nurses: Implications for primary care. *Policy, Politics, & Nursing Practice, 11,* 89–98.

Delgado-Passler, P., & McCaffrey, R. (2006). The influences of postdischarge management by nurse practitioners on hospital readmission for heart failure. *Journal of the American Academy of Nurse Practitioners, 18,* 154–160.

Edmunds, M. (2001). Why don't we receive equal reimbursement? *Nurse Practitioner.* Retrieved from http://findarticles.com/p/articles/mi_qa3958/is_200212/ai_ n9164785/?tag=rbxcra.2.a.11

Evans, T., & Frakes, M. A. (2006). An overview of Medicare reimbursement regulations for advanced practice nurses. *Nursing Economics, 24*(2), 59–65. Retrieved from http://www.medscape.com/viewarticle/531035

Gosfield, A. G. (2001). The ins and outs of "incident-to" reimbursement. *Family Practice Management, 23–27.*

Hull-Grommesh, L., Ellis, E. F., & Mackey, T. A. (2010). Implications for cardiology nurse practitioner billing: A comparison of hospital versus office practice. *Journal of the American Academy of Nurse Practitioners, 22,* 288–291.

Institute of Medicine. (2011). *The future of nursing: Leading change, advancing health.* Washington, DC: The National Academies Press.

Jacobs, P. (1996). *The economics of health and medical care* (4th ed.). Gaithersburg, MD: Aspen.

Lee, S. (2011). In support of the abolishment of supervisory and collaboration clauses. *Journal for Nurse Practitioners, 7,* 764–769.

Mezey, M., Burger, S. G., Bloom, H. G., Bonner, A., Bourbonniere, M., Bowers, B., & Dimant, J. (2005). Experts recommend strategies for strengthening the use of advanced practice nurses in nursing homes. *Journal of the American Geriatrics Society, 53,* 1790–1797.

O'Brien, S. (2011). *Baby boomers and healthcare: What are the problems, and what can be done?* Retrieved from http://seniorliving.about.com/od/manageyourmoney/a/ healthcarecosts.htm

O'Grady, E. T. & Brassard, A. (2011). Health-care reform: Opportunities for NPs and urgency for modernizing nurse practice acts. *Journal of Nursing Regulation, 2,* 4–9.

QFinance. (2011). *Understanding economic efficiency theory.* Retrieved from http://www .qfinance.com/corporate-governance-checklists/understanding-economic-efficiency- theory

Sullivan-Marx, E. M. (2008). Lessons learned from advanced practice nursing payment. *Policy, Politics and Nursing Practice, 9,* 121–126.

Weiland, S. A. (2008). Reflections on independence in nurse practitioner practice. *Journal of the American Academy of Nurse Practitioners, 20,* 345–352.

Wilensky, G. R. (2009). Reforming Medicare's physician payment system. *New England Journal of Medicine, 360,* 653–655. Retrieved from http://www.nejm.org/doi/ full/10.1056/NEJMp0808003

Zhang, N. J., Unruh, L., & Wan, T. T. (2008). Has the Medicare prospective payment system led to increased nursing home efficiency? *Health Services Research, 43*(3), 1043–1061.

10

Enhancement of Neonatal Hypothermia Prevention and Recognition Skills in Rural Uganda

Elizabeth Whitworth and Barbara A. Anderson

DNP Essential #6
Interprofessional collaboration for improving patient and population health outcomes

American Association of Colleges of Nursing. (2006). *The essentials of doctoral education for advanced nursing practice.* Retrieved from http://www.aacn.nche.edu/publications/position/DNPEssentials.pdf

This chapter describes cross-cultural collaboration in decreasing risk for adverse outcomes related to neonatal hypothermia among Ugandan neonates.

It exemplifies DNP *Essential #6* as it relates to both collaboration and to improving health outcomes.

The capstone demonstrates sustainability as demonstrated by cultural assimilation and integration into existing clinical practices. It has potential for replicability with minimal cost in low-resource settings.

Barbara A. Anderson, Editor

CAPSTONE FOCUS

Catastrophic events, such as armed conflict, displacement of persons from conflict areas, genocide, epidemics, famine, malnutrition, lack of basic resources, and natural disasters quickly overwhelm health care systems. The decades-long, ongoing conflict in northern Uganda, East Africa, has put enormous pressure on existing health care systems, decreasing access to care for both local tribal populations and displaced persons migrating from conflict areas. Pregnant women and their infants have been particularly vulnerable. This capstone project targeted potentially life-threatening hypothermia among newborns in the Teso region of rural, eastern Uganda.

REVIEW OF THE LITERATURE

Each year 2 million newborns die within 24 hours of birth (United Nations Population Fund [UNFPA], 2011). Of the 3.7 million neonatal deaths and 3.3 million stillbirths each year, 98% occur in developing countries (Carlo et al., 2010).

Neonatal Hypothermia

Neonatal hypothermia has been well documented throughout the developing world as an important source of neonatal morbidity, but is not a commonly recognized threat to neonatal well-being (Carlo et al., 2010). Neonatal hypothermia is defined by the World Health Organization (WHO) as a core body temperature of less than 36.5 degrees Celsius (97.7 degrees Fahrenheit; WHO, 1997). In low-resource settings in developing countries, hypothermia at birth is one of the most important risk factors for morbidity and mortality in newborn infants of all birth weights and gestational ages (Wariki & Mori, 2010; WHO, 1997).

Sobel, Silvestre, Mantaring, Oliveros, and Nyunt-U (2011) found that unmitigated hypothermia poses serious threats to newborns, including respiratory distress syndrome, delayed fetal-to-newborn circulatory transition, coagulation defects, acidosis, infection, and brain hemorrhage. Baghban, Jambarsang, Pezeshk, and Nayeri (2012) found that prolonged hypothermia is associated with increased risk of cold injury manifested by symptoms including lethargy; a slowing heart rate corresponding to decreased body temperature; and slow, shallow, irregular respirations. Pulmonary hemorrhage, acidemia, jaundice, and hypoglycemia are consequences associated with prolonged neonatal hypothermia (Zayeri, Kazemnejad, Ganjali, Babaei, & Nayeri, 2007). Excess mortality is extended beyond the neonatal period into the second month of life by a single episode of neonatal hypothermia (Sodemann et al., 2008).

Recognition of Hypothermia by Health Care Providers

Health care providers may fail to recognize and treat early symptoms of neonatal hypothermia due to lack of knowledge or inadequate equipment for hypothermia detection (Kumar, Shearer, Kumar, & Darmstadt, 2009). Choudbury, Bajaj, and Gupta (2000) identified a significant knowledge deficit in hypothermia management among health care providers in low-resource settings and recommended enhanced training in order to reduce neonatal mortality and morbidity. Regardless of etiology, prevention, and management of neonatal hypothermia, it can potentially lower neonatal mortality by 18% to 24% (Darmstadt et al., 2005).

Prevention and Management of Neonatal Thermoregulation

The WHO (1997) has practice guidelines for the prevention and management of neonatal hypothermia. These guidelines, the *warm chain,* are 10 interrelated steps to be taken at birth and in the following hours and days to prevent and manage neonatal hypothermia. These steps include: warm delivery room, immediate drying, skin-to-skin contact, immediate breastfeeding, postponement of bathing and weighing, appropriate clothing/bedding, keeping mother and baby together, warm transportation, warm resuscitation, and enhanced training. Failure to implement any of the links in the warm chain increases risk for hypothermia development.

There is abundant evidence that supports widespread implementation of these steps. Immediate skin-to-skin placement of the newborn and the mother has been well researched as a positive measure to prevent and manage neonatal hypothermia (Bergstrom, Okong, & Ransjo-Arvidson, 2007; DiMenna, 2006; Galligan, 2006; Mullany, 2010; Sobel et al., 2011). Close body contact between mother and infant immediately after birth supports not only newborn temperature regulation, but also energy conservation, acid-base balance, adjustment of respiration, crying, and positive breastfeeding behaviors (Winberg, 2005).

In a systematic review, Puig and Sguassero (2007) found that skin-to-skin contact between the mother and newborn immediately after birth reduces crying, improves mother-infant interaction, keeps the baby warm, and facilitates breastfeeding. A systematic review among diverse populations in Canada, Chile, Guatemala, Israel, Japan, Nepal, Poland, Russia, South Africa, Spain, Sweden, Taiwan, Thailand, the United Kingdom, and the United States examined the effect of early skin-to-skin contact on breastfeeding, maternal and infant behavior, and physiological adaptation in healthy mother-newborn dyads. The findings identified a statistically significant increase in the ability of skin-to-skin contact infants to maintain stable temperatures in the neutral thermal range (Moore, Anderson, & Bergman, 2009).

Neonatal Hypothermia in Uganda

Uganda is predominantly rural, with a high fertility rate, low contraception use and availability, and one of the fastest-growing populations in the world. The maternal mortality ratio is 430 per 100,000 live births and neonatal mortality rate is 31 per 1,000 live births. Ugandan women have a 1 in 35 lifetime risk of maternal death related to pregnancy and childbearing, with 42% of births attended by skilled health personnel (United Nations Population Fund [UNFPA], 2011).

Neonatal hypothermia is a serious newborn problem in Uganda. Bergstrom, Byaruhanga, and Okong (2004) found that up to 80% of newborns suffered from hypothermia within the first hour after birth. A study in a periurban hospital in Kampala, Uganda, Byaruhanga, Bergstrom, and Okong (2005) observed lack of newborn skin-to-skin contact with mothers among 87% of hypothermic newborns. Location in a hospital in a tropical setting, with room temperatures ranging between 20 and 27 degrees Celsius (68 to 80.6 degrees Fahrenheit), was not found to preclude the occurrence of neonatal hypothermia. The authors concluded that protocols promoting skin-to-skin contact to promote thermoregulation were not routinely implemented, nor was skin-to-skin contact an accepted cultural norm. Ahmed et al. (2011) drew similar conclusions, finding that mothers who were taught skin-to-skin practices did so in a token manner unlikely to improve health or survival. Widespread cultural acceptance of skin-to-skin practices remains an elusive issue in Uganda.

The Midwifery Handbook and Guide to Practice, endorsed by the Ugandan Ministry of Health, includes specific guidelines for immediate placement of the newborn on the mother's abdomen, early initiation of breastfeeding, and keeping the newborn dry and warm (Uganda Nurse and Midwives Council, 2001). While endorsing this midwifery document and identifying improved newborn care as a priority in national health policy, there is no provision by the Ministry of Health to monitor or enforce compliance to the guidelines. Waisa et al. (2010) concluded that health care providers practicing in underserved regions of the country lacked adequate knowledge and skills in keeping the newborn warm and in promoting early breastfeeding as a thermoregulatory measure.

THE CAPSTONE PROJECT

Prior to the initiation of this capstone project, I volunteered at a clinic sponsored by a nongovernmental organization in the Teso region of rural, eastern Uganda. The Teso region is a high plateau encircled by mountains. The climate is tropical, warm, rainy, and humid. The widespread prevalence of malaria, minimal infrastructure, lack of access to clean drinking water, and frequent electricity outages are serious challenges encountered in this setting.

Description of the Clinic

The clinic, which includes a birth facility, offers comprehensive medical services to vulnerable and destitute populations in the Teso region, as well as refugees who have relocated from conflict regions in northern Uganda. The clinic is a rented, concrete block building located on an unpaved road in a residential area and is staffed by Ugandan *comprehensive* nurses who have received training beyond basic nursing in specialty areas including midwifery.

Early each morning, patients and families arrive at the clinic by foot, bicycle, or *bajaj*, local motorcycles for hire. The clinic has limited funds for reimbursing bajaj drivers who bring women in labor from outlying villages. The waiting room is an open-air setting with wooden benches and a tin roof covering a concrete slab. The clinic day begins with songful prayer expressing gratitude for the day, blessings received, and services to be rendered followed by general announcements to the patients about clinic operations and protocol. A clinic appointment is an all-day affair, with registration, history taking, vital signs, examination, procedures, laboratory tests, pharmacy, immunizations, and discharge teaching. All services are provided free of charge with no criteria for eligibility.

When a woman presents for evaluation of labor, she is escorted to the birth room. She climbs on a step stool onto the labor bed, a hospital gurney covered with a sheet of black plastic. The birth center has no provision for linens, sheets, receiving blankets, sanitary napkins, or laundry. A *birth kit* consists of a pair of sterile gloves, sterilized scissors, bulb syringe, and string to ligate the umbilical cord. If delivery is not imminent, the laboring mother is encouraged to walk the clinic grounds and eat and drink. Patients and their families are expected to bring their own provisions and have access to untreated tap water and outdoor latrines. It is not an uncommon occurrence for the family of a laboring mother to set up a small camp with a cooking fire near the clinic grounds.

When she thinks delivery is imminent, the laboring mother returns to the birthing room and climbs onto the gurney where the birth is attended by a comprehensive nurse. Although the comprehensive nurse has not completed a full specialist course in midwifery, she has completed a multi-skilled training course including basic midwifery skills.

Once delivered, the newborn is briefly dried with cloth supplied by the mother. The nurse cuts the cord and the infant is placed across the room from the mother. There is no *warming bed* for the newborn and limited resources for infant resuscitation. Even if full-blown resuscitation were possible, there is limited availability of neonatal intensive care in a referral hospital. The primary emphasis in the clinic is on safe motherhood and caring for the mother, as her loss or incapacitation would be devastating to her husband and often leave numerous children at home to fend for themselves. Once the mother has been stabilized and evaluated, the newborn is weighed, examined, and receives a vitamin K injection and antibiotic eye prophylaxis. The mother is then bathed and escorted to the postpartum ward where she is reunited with her newborn and encouraged to breastfeed.

One of the practices that made the deepest impression on me was the routine practice of immediately cutting the umbilical cord and physically separating the newborn away from its mother. As a midwife who has practiced in home birth, birth center, and high- and low-risk hospital settings, I brought significant prior experience in examining a range of practices related to the timing of cord clamping and infant placement after birth. I remember feeling compelled to repeatedly walk over to where the infant lay, reassuring myself the newborn was alive and breathing. I noted that the newborns were generally less vigorous than the lusty babies to whom I had grown accustomed in my practice. Due to the setting and circumstance of their births, these newborns encountered challenges that put them at particular risk for issues related to heat loss and thermoregulation, increasing the risk for neonatal hypothermia.

Development of the Project

Leininger's Transcultural Nursing Theory guided the planning and implementation of my DNP capstone project. The central purpose of this theory is discovery and explanation of culturally based factors that influence the health, well-being, illness, and death of vulnerable populations (Leininger, 2002). The goal is to provide safe care within a culturally congruent environment. Culturally congruent care fits the existing value system and life patterns, and is not based on predetermined criteria. Culturally competent care requires the practitioner to bridge cultural gaps in providing supportive and meaningful care without imposition of one's own beliefs, practices, and values (Current Nursing, 2012).

Leininger contends that discordance between the generic or folk care practices (emic) and biomedical (etic) practices may result in care that is not culturally congruent (Zoucha, 2012). To provide culturally congruent care, Leininger proposes a bridge between emic and etic systems. Grounded in both emic and etic knowledge, three predictive modes of action may inform and describe the delivery of culturally congruent and beneficial care: 1) culture care preservation and/or maintenance, 2) culture care accommodation and/or negotiation, and 3) culture care repatterning and/or restructuring (Current Nursing, 2012).

The goal of my DNP Capstone Project was to collaborate with the clinic staff in the design and implementation of a culturally congruent education program to decrease the risk for neonatal hypothermia. Wherever possible, cultural practices were acknowledged, validated, and retained. Based upon evidence-based practices for neonatal hypothermia prevention, this project targeted skin-to-skin care as a low-technology clinical intervention that could potentially be accommodated in the clinic birth culture. The American College of Nurse-Midwives Life-Saving Skills series (Buffington, Beck, & Clark, 2008) was a foundational document in the development of the plan, and I was privileged to have Sandra Buffington as a member of my capstone committee.

Implementation of the Project

Project implementation occurred over a designated 4-week period. The initial step was administration of a pretest to the comprehensive nursing staff to determine baseline knowledge about neonatal hypothermia. A spirited group discussion of cultural beliefs and practices followed. The goals and purpose of the education program were introduced. The staff was invited to describe the current newborn care practices, their perceptions of the influence of belief systems and culture, and the rationale for these practices. Sometimes it was something as simple as "that is the way it has always been done." Other times it was something that I, as an outsider from a different cultural perspective, might not have considered.

The birth center staff identified cultural fear and aversion to contact with body fluids among the mothers. The staff also expressed a belief that hypothermia was not likely to occur in tropical settings, but conceded it was possible and wanted to provide the most appropriate care. Planning and implementation was adapted as much as possible to address these beliefs and values. Further, the birth center staff expressed value for skin-to-skin practices as a measure to prevent or manage hypothermia, although they lacked skills in hypothermia management. The staff offered ideas on facilitating cultural acceptance and assimilation of skin-to-skin care into practice.

Weeks 2 and 3 consisted of planned educational program sessions. The concept of evidence-based practices as the foundation for best practices in the clinical setting was presented. A summary of the literature supporting skin-to-skin practices as evidence-based included the existence of neonatal hypothermia as a valid threat to newborn well-being, signs and symptoms of its development and occurrence, ensuing short- and long-term consequences, and prevention measures.

During Week 2, staff collaborated using their artistic and linguistic abilities to assist with creation of posters, in English as well as the two prevalent tribal languages, Atesot and Kuman. A theme, *everyone wins with skin-to-skin,* was created and utilized as a visual reminder for staff and for purposes of introducing the neonatal hypothermia prevention measures concept to the patient population. The posters were displayed in prominent locations in the clinic, the birth room, and the postpartum ward.

During Week 3, multiple sessions were offered to allow skills demonstration and practice sessions. During these sessions, staff members were provided the opportunity to engage in key learning point discussions, practice, and perform skills until they self-identified mastery. The next step was discussion of problematic situations and how to problem solve, especially related to assimilation of skin-to-skin practices into current practice routines. The group consensus was that introduction of the concept of hypothermia prevention measures and practices during antenatal clinic and again during labor prior to delivery would increase acceptance of skin-to-skin practices by the women giving birth.

Evaluation of the education program occurred in the final week through a written posttest, shared verbal knowledge, and a return skills demonstration. The opportunity to verbalize educational content learned, rather than relying solely on pre- and posttest scores, was included in the evaluation process as an added measure for evaluation of participants who could potentially have been unfamiliar with pre- and posttest formats. Fortunately, no such difficulty was encountered. All of the comprehensive nursing staff participated in the education program activities, including baseline pretest, discussion of cultural beliefs and practices, education sessions, poster creation, and evaluation activities. There was a statistically significant increase in both knowledge and skills in the prevention and management of neonatal hypothermia among all of the participants ($p = .011$). All participants reported that this educational project enhanced their skills in neonatal hypothermia prevention, recognition, and management.

IMPACT

Skin-to-skin care as a neonatal hypothermia prevention measure is endorsed and supported by both the Ugandan Nurse and Midwives Council and Ugandan Ministry of Health (Uganda Nurse and Midwives Council, 2001). Collaboration with the comprehensive nursing staff and their unqualified enthusiasm and support were essential to promoting skin-to-skin care. This project was a collaborative effort to craft a culturally sensitive, participative education program for comprehensive nursing staff members, aiming to provide multiple culturally appropriate opportunities for knowledge acquisition and demonstration of learning objectives.

Perhaps the most rewarding moment of this project occurred when I was greeted one morning by a well-respected nursing staff member exclaiming, "It works; it really works!" He described the common perception that Ugandan newborns are quiet and calm by nature. He then related how he had implemented skin-to-skin practices at deliveries over the night and experienced uncharacteristically loud and vigorous protests from the infants when they were finally separated from their mothers for weighing and examination.

While this represents a simple continuing education project in one low-resource and conflict-ridden region, it is significant because it empowered the comprehensive nursing staff to participate actively in prevention of one of the most easily preventable causes of neonatal mortality and morbidity in low-resource areas. Positive outcomes associated with the educational project include demonstrated increased staff provider knowledge. There is also potential for overall improved perinatal outcomes, decreased hospital transfers, and decreased family and institutional debt. Moreover, there is the potential for a change in the routine standard of care at the birth center, incorporating evidence-based skin-to-skin practices, increased cultural acceptance of skin-to-skin practices, and avoidance of long-term health consequences associated with neonatal hypothermia.

There is much potential for broader application and impact in future expansion operations. Serendipity in this project was the opportunity to improve outcomes in the outlying villages. The clinic operates a mobile outreach clinic one day per week, providing care to pregnant women in remote villages who often live too far away to come to the birth center. Teaching skin-to-skin practices in the outreach clinic setting for births occurring in the home is an example of program expansion that is simple to implement and requires no additional resources. This learning integration has the potential to impact population health, especially among the most vulnerable and underserved in rural Uganda.

REFERENCES

Ahmed, S., Mitra, S. N., Chowdbury, A. M., Camacho, L. L., Winikoff, B., & Sloan, N. L. (2011). Community kangaroo mother care: Implementation and potential for neonatal survival and health in very low-income settings. *Journal of Perinatology, 31*(5), 361–367. doi:10.1038/jp.2010.131

American College of Nurse–Midwives. (2008). *Life-saving skills manual for midwives* (4th ed.). Silver Spring, MD: Author.

Baghban, A. A., Jambarsang, S., Pezeshk, H., & Nayeri, F. (2012). The effects of temperature and birth weight on the transition rate of hypothermia in hospitalized neonates using Markov models. *Tehran University Medical Journal, 70*(5), 282–288.

Bergstrom, A., Byaruhanga, R., & Okong, P. (2004). Comparison of tympanic and rectal thermometry: Diagnosis of neonatal hypothermia in Uganda. *Journal of Neonatal Nursing, 10*(1), 6–9.

Bergstrom, A., Okong, P., & Ransjo-Arvidson, A. (2007). Immediate maternal thermal response to skin-to-skin care of newborn. *Acta Paediatrica, 96*(5), 655–658. doi:10.1111/j.1651-2227.2007.00280.x

Byaruhanga, R., Bergstrom, A., & Okong, P. (2005). Neonatal hypothermia in Uganda: Prevalence and risk factors. *Journal of Tropical Pediatrics, 51*(4), 212–215.

Carlo, W., Goudar, S., Jehan, I., Chomba, E., Tshefu, A., Garces, A., . . . Wright, L. L. (2010). Newborn-care training and perinatal mortality in developing countries. *New England Journal of Medicine, 362*(7), 614–623. doi:10.1056/NEJMsa0806033

Choudbury, S. P., Bajaj, R. K., & Gupta, R. K. (2000). Knowledge, attitude and practices about neonatal hypothermia among medical and paramedical staff. *Indian Journal of Pediatrics, 67*(7), 491–496.

Current Nursing. (2012). *Transcultural nursing.* Retrieved from http://currentnursing.com/nursing_theory/transcultural_nursing.html

Darmstadt, G., Bhutta, Z., Cousens, S., Adam, T., Walker, N., & de Bernis, L. (2005). Evidence-based, cost-effective interventions: How many newborn babies can we save? *Lancet, 365*(9463), 977–988.

DiMenna, L. (2006). Considerations for implementation of a neonatal kangaroo care protocol. *Neonatal Network, 25*(6), 405–412.

Galligan, M. (2006). Proposed guidelines for skin-to-skin treatment of neonatal hypothermia. *The American Journal of Maternal Child Nursing, 31*(5), 298–304.

Kumar, V., Shearer, J. C., Kumar, A., & Darmstadt, G. L. (2009). Neonatal hypothermia in low resource settings: A review. *Journal of Perinatology, 29*(6), 401–412. doi:10.1038/jp.2008.233

Leininger, M. (2002). Culture care theory: A major contribution to advance transcultural nursing knowledge and practices. *Journal of Transcultural Nursing, 13*(3), 189–192.

Moore, E. R., Anderson, G. C., & Bergman, N. (2009). Early skin-to-skin contact for mothers and their healthy newborn infants. *Cochrane Database Systematic Reviews,* (1). doi:10.1002/14651858.CD003519

Mullany, L. (2010). Neonatal hypothermia in low-resource settings. *Seminars in Perinatology, 34*(6), 426–433. doi:10.1053/j.semperi.2010.09.007

Puig, G., & Sguassero, Y. (2007, November 9). *Early skin-to-skin contact for mothers and their healthy newborn infants: RHL commentary.* Retrieved from http://apps.who.int/rhl/archives/gpcom/en/index.html

Sobel, H. L., Silvestre, M. A., Mantaring, J. B., III, Oliveros, Y. E., & Nyunt-U, S. (2011). Immediate newborn care practices delay thermoregulation and breastfeeding initiation. *Acta Paediatrica, 100*(8), 1127–1133. doi:10.1111/j.1651-2227.2011.02215.x

Sodemann, M., Nielsen, J., Veirum, J., Jakobsen, M. S., Biai, S., & Aaby, P. (2008). Hypothermia of newborns is associated with excess mortality in the first 2 months of life in Guineau-Bissau, West Africa. *Tropical Medicine and International Health, 13*(8), 980–986. doi:10.1111/j.1365-3156.2008.02113.x

Uganda Nurse and Midwives Council. (2001). *Midwifery handbook and guide to practice* (11th ed.). Kampala, Uganda: Ugandan Ministry of Health.

United Nations Population Fund. (2011). *The state of the world's midwifery 2011: Delivering health, saving lives.* Retrieved from www.stateoftheworldsmidwifery.com

Waisa, P., Nyanzi, S., Namusoko-Kalungi, S., Peterson, S., Tomson, G., & Pariyo, G. W. (2010). I never thought that this baby would survive; I thought that it would die any time: Perceptions and care for preterm babies in eastern Uganda. *Tropical Medicine and International Health, 15*(10), 1140–1147. doi:10.1111/j.1365-3156.2010.02603.x

Wariki, W. M., & Mori, R. (2010, June 1). *Interventions to prevent hypothermia at birth in preterm and/or low-birth-weight infants: RHL commentary.* Retrieved from http://apps.who.int/rhl/newborn/cd004210_Warikiwmv_com/en/index.html

Winberg, J. (2005). Mother and newborn baby: Mutual regulation of physiology and behavior—A selective review. *Developmental Psychobiology, 47*(3), 217–229.

World Health Organization. (1997). *Thermal protection of the newborn: A practical guide.* Retrieved from http://whqlibdoc.who.int/hq/1997/WHO_RHT_MSM_97.2.pdf

Zayeri, F., Kazemnejad, A., Ganjali, M., Babaei, G., & Nayeri, F. (2007). Incidence and risk factors of neonatal hypothermia at referral hospitals in Tehran, Islamic Republic of Iran. *Eastern Mediterranean Health Journal, 13*(6), 1308–1318.

Zoucha, R. (2012). The utility of Leininger's culture care theory with vulnerable populations. In M. de Chesnay & B. A. Anderson (Eds.), *Caring for the vulnerable: Perspectives in nursing theory, practice, and research* (3rd ed., pp. 147–152). Burlington, MA: Jones & Bartlett.

11

Hypertension Group Health Care Visits: Improving Clinical Outcomes

Heather Shlosser and Edie Devers Barbero

DNP Essential #7

**Clinical prevention and population health
for improving the nation's health**

American Association of Colleges of Nursing. (2006). *The essentials of doctoral education for advanced nursing practice.* Retrieved from http://www.aacn.nche.edu/publications/position/DNPEssentials.pdf

This chapter describes the development of group health care visits to manage hypertension. The project was a systems change from the current individual primary care treatment of hypertension to a group model that included clinical management, psychological support, and information to improve hypertension control.

It exemplifies DNP *Essential #7* as it relates to clinical prevention and improving health.

Joyce M. Knestrick, Editor

CAPSTONE FOCUS

There has been a steady increase in hypertension awareness, prevention, treatment, and control over the past 10 years (Yoon, Burt, Louis, & Carroll, 2012). Yet hypertension remains epidemic and one of the most common reasons for primary care visits, with an estimated 46.3 million visits per year (Schappert & Rechtsteiner, 2011). Successful management requires a comprehensive approach, including access to care, prevention and treatment services, and patient awareness and compliance (Centers for Disease Control and Prevention [CDC], 2011).

This capstone project addressed these elements of management by implementing a clinical practice change from individual primary care to holistic, preventive care within a group setting for patients with hypertension. The organization framework for this capstone was Wagner's Chronic Care Model (CCM), incorporating clinical management, psychological support, and information essential for identification and improved control of hypertension (Wagner et al., 2001).

REVIEW OF THE LITERATURE

The Scope of the Problem

According to the *Seventh Report of the Joint National Committee on Prevention, Detection, Evaluation, and Treatment of High Blood Pressure* (United States Department of Health and Human Services [USDHHS], 2004), blood pressure greater than 120/80 is defined as prehypertension and blood pressure higher than 140/90 is defined as clinical hypertension. Data from the CDC (2011) estimate that 1 in 3 adults are hypertensive, which equates to an estimated 68 million Americans. In the United States, hypertension is responsible for 35% of all cardiovascular events, 49% of all episodes of heart failure, and 24% of all premature deaths (Sheridan, Pignone, & Donahue, 2003). Effective intervention and treatment of hypertension is required to avoid potential adverse outcomes such as myocardial infarction, stroke, heart failure, or renal failure (Ong, Cheung, Man, Lau, & Lam, 2007). Yet it is estimated that only 50% of patients diagnosed with hypertension have sufficiently controlled blood pressures (Yoon et al., 2012).

Data from the *National Health and Nutrition Examination Survey (NHANES III;* Wang & Wang, 2004) reported that among 16,095 adults:

- 32% were unaware of being hypertensive and were not receiving treatment
- 15% were aware of their diagnosis but were not receiving treatment
- 26% were receiving treatment but continued to have uncontrolled hypertension
- 27% were treated and were subsequently normotensive

Further, 66% of patients with hypertension were not advised by their health care providers to institute lifestyle modifications or start pharmacological interventions (Wang & Wang, 2004).

Causes for Poor Outcomes

Inadequate knowledge and/or noncompliance among patients and the lack of a caring, therapeutic partnership with a health provider are two reasons associated with poor blood pressure control (Mohammadi, Abedi, Gofranipour, & Jalali, 2002). Time constraints placed upon primary care providers are a significant barrier to the development of a therapeutic relationship. Ostby et al.

(2005) reviewed the care for 2,500 primary care patients with poor chronic care management, examining time constraints among providers as a possible cause of inadequate chronic care management. The researchers calculated the effect of disease control status on time requirements for 10 combined chronic conditions, including hyperlipidemia, hypertension, depression, asthma, diabetes, arthritis, anxiety, osteoporosis, chronic obstructive pulmonary disease, and coronary artery disease. The amount of time required to provide high-quality, comprehensive, guideline-based care exceeded the time allotment to providers for all patient care.

Group Visits as a Strategy for Chronic Care Management

To address time constraints in the primary care setting, group visits have been suggested as a way to promote more patient–provider interaction, education, evaluation, treatment planning, and follow-up care (Jaber, Braksmajer, & Trilling, 2006a). In a systematic review of group visits published from 1974 to 2004, Jaber et al. (2006a) concluded that ". . . group visits improved patient and physician satisfaction, quality of care, and quality of life, as well as decrease health care utilization" (p. 288). Edelman et al. (2010) conducted a randomized trial of 239 patients with hypertension and diabetes to examine the impact of group visits on blood pressure control and A1c. Patients in group visit settings have been found to have greater blood pressure control compared to individual care.

Group visits are generally 2 hours in length and permit for greater time between patient and provider. The group has at least one physician, nurse practitioner (NP), or physician assistant who may or may not be the group facilitator. There is generally support staff managing the clinic flow for check in and out, vital signs, medication reconciliation, follow-up plan confirmation, and data entry in the electronic medical record (Abramowitz, Flattery, Franses, & Berry, 2010; Houck, Kilo, & Scott, 2003; Jaber, Braksmajer, & Trilling, 2006b).

Organizational Support

Implementing group visits in the clinical setting requires organizational support (Jaber et al., 2006a, 2006b). Group visit programs are time intensive and require administrative support because of financial implications, allocation of human resources, and physical space. Patient recruitment, registration, program design and structure, developing the interdisciplinary team, supplies, pre- and postvisit preparation, supplies, tracking quality improvement, and outcome evaluation are all tied to administrative support (Wagner et al., 2001). Consensus among providers across the health system also enhances the potential for success and sustainability of the program.

Venue for Patient Education

Group visits are not only a logical venue for supportive interaction among patients, but also provide opportunity for education as well as a forum for history taking, vital signs, physical assessment, treatment planning, and follow-up. Group health care visits allow for specialist guest speakers, community connections, peer-to-peer interaction, and focus on clinical prevention and lifestyle modification. Topics can be provider or patient driven but generally include medication management, stress management and coping skills, nutrition, exercise, and community resources—all with a primary focus on enhanced prevention and self-management. As providers often struggle with responding to patients who experience difficulty with self-management skills such as goal setting, personal action plans, or support for failed plans, the group visit approach is a model with great potential for helping patients with self-management skills (Abramowitz et al., 2010; Houck et al., 2003; Jaber et al., 2006b).

Billing for Group Visits

There is no optimum way to bill for group visits, a key aspect in implementing this model (Jaber et al., 2006b). However, organizations that take a broader look at the financial and quality-of-care outcomes, beyond running the program, can expect to offset annual per-patient costs accrued in emergency room visits and unplanned office visits from patients with uncontrolled hypertension. In 2009, approximately 56.5 million individuals or 24.4% of adults age 18 and older had some health care expenses for hypertension (Davis, 2012). Direct medical spending to treat hypertension equaled $47.5 billion in 2009, with almost half ($21.4 billion) in the form of prescription medications (Davis, 2012). In the randomized trial conducted by Edelman et al. (2010), the average per-patient annual cost for group visit participation including follow-up phone calls was $460. With an annual per-patient reduction of 0.4 emergency department visits and 0.9 primary care visits among group visit participants, the per patient cost of $460 is a significant offset.

THE CAPSTONE PROJECT

Project Design

This capstone project utilized a quasiexperimental, nonequivalent control group pretest-posttest design to test the hypotheses that participation in group visits would demonstrate (1) decreased blood pressure readings and (2) increased self-efficacy scores compared to those patients who received care individually. The independent variable was the group visit intervention. The dependent variables were blood pressure and self-efficacy scores. Blood pressure was measured with a standard blood pressure cuff. The measure of self-efficacy was The Stanford Patient Education Research Center Self-Efficacy for Managing Chronic Disease 6-Item Scale Questions (see Figure 11.1). This study was conducted in the worksite primary care clinic of a large grocery distributor corporation serving approximately 3,000 employees and their family members from ages 2 years onward. Such a setting has inherent time constraints on employee participation in group health programs. In addition, if employees left the corporation, they were no longer eligible for services within the health center.

After review of data from the clinic's electronic health record, 193 patients were found to have diagnosed hypertension. Participants were recruited from the eligible worksite clinic population, which resulted in a sample from the

FIGURE 11.1 *Stanford Patient Education Research Center Self-Efficacy for Managing Chronic Disease 6-Item Scale Questions*

Self-Efficacy for Managing Chronic Disease 6-Item Scale

1. How confident are you that you can keep the fatigue caused by your disease from interfering with the things you want to do?

2. How confident are you that you can keep the physical discomfort or pain of your disease from interfering with the things you want to do?

3. How confident are you that you can keep the emotional distress caused by your disease from interfering with the things you want to do?

4. How confident are you that you can keep any other symptoms or health problems you have from interfering with the things you want to do?

5. How confident are you that you can do the different tasks and activities needed to manage your health condition so as to reduce your need to see a doctor?

6. How confident are you that you can do things other than just taking medication to reduce how much your illness affects your everyday life?

Adapted from Stanford Patient Education Center, Stanford School of Medicine (2014).

community and from multiple primary care provider practices. Recruitment included mailings and phone calls to patients listed in the high-risk disease management hypertension database. E-mail invitations were sent out through the corporation's intranet and the patient health care portal. The initial sample for the study was 30 participants. Two participants dropped out of the program, yielding a final sample of 28. The treatment group and the comparison group each consisted of 14 participants. See Table 11.1 for the description of the participants.

For the intervention group, group visits included group education and interaction and most elements of an individual patient visit, including collection of vital signs, history taking, and brief system-specific physical exam. The educational aspect of the program included interactive discussions related to how to attain optimally controlled blood pressure. The program incorporated usual hypertension care and education and expanded education on nutrition, cardiopulmonary exercise options, mind/body education, meditation sessions, and stress management. Any recommended medication changes were reviewed with the patient's primary care provider. There were no medication changes made in the intervention group during the study period. Three out of 14 comparison group participants had their hypertension medication increased during the 12-week study period.

The intervention group, those engaged in group health visits, met for a 3-month time period with a total of four group visit sessions. The comparison group, those receiving treatment as usual from an NP, were followed with

TABLE 11.1 *Characteristics of Participants*

	Intervention Group Group Visit (*n* = 14)	Comparison Group Treatment as Usual (*n* = 14)
Age		
Gender	52.5	42.14
Male	5	10
Female	9	4
Race		
Black	1	0
White (non-Hispanic)	11	13
Indian	2	1
Primary care provider		
Yes	13	13
No	1	1
# of hypertension medications		
1 medication	7	8
2 medications	7	6
Smoker	2	2
Nonsmoker	12	12

evidenced-based hypertension guidelines in a primary care clinic setting during the same 3-month period.

Each participant began the program with a 1:1 individual visit with the NP to obtain informed consent for participation prior to starting the program. Participants in the intervention group had fasting biometrics and the *Stanford Self-Efficacy Assessment* completed prior to participating in the group intervention (time point 1) and following completion of the program (time point 2). Participants in the comparison group had fasting biometrics and the self-efficacy assessment completed at the same time periods as the intervention group. All participants were offered ongoing health coaching at the conclusion of the program as well as a refresher drop-in group visit over the following year.

Ethical Considerations

Institutional review board (IRB) approval was obtained from the University of Virginia Health Systems. Patients who registered for the study signed an informed consent form prior to participation in the program, and patients with primary care providers were requested to sign an additional consent to release information to their primary care provider. Clinic staff informed the participants' primary care providers via form letter that their patients had registered for participation in the program. Upon culmination of the program, a final summary was sent to the primary care providers, informing them of the overall program results in addition to the individual patient biometrics results and blood pressure readings.

CASE STUDY PART I

**Mrs. J: A Patient With Hypertension
and Other Chronic Illnesses**

Mrs. J is a 52-year-old female patient. She presented to the wellness center reporting, "I just don't feel healthy and I am frustrated that I don't know what to do about it." Mrs. J reported she was feeling "tired all the time and very unmotivated to make any changes." She felt "bounced around" the health care system and never felt like she is being heard in her "10- to 15-minute visits." She was being followed by her primary care provider, a cardiologist, and an endocrinologist. She had uncontrolled type 2 hypertension, type 2 diabetes, hyperlipidemia, depression, asthma, and obesity. At the time she presented to the wellness center she was taking amlodipine and lisinopril for her hypertension; metformin for her diabetes; pravastatin for her hyperlipidemia; Flovent, Proair, Zyrtec, and Flonase for her asthma and allergies; citalopram for her depression; fish oil; and a multivitamin "because my doctor told me I should."

Mrs. J is a nonsmoker and does not use any alcohol or illicit drugs. She takes her medications as directed; however, does not feel they are "helping at all." She has a poor diet and confirms that she is an "emotional eater." She eats fast food frequently, frozen foods, and does not eat many fruits or vegetables. She does not exercise, and considers herself to be a "couch potato" because she "wouldn't know where to start" with an exercise program or more active lifestyle. She is married in a mutually monogamous relationship free of physical abuse. She does not feel well supported by her husband. She works full-time and feels some of her coworkers would be a good source of support if she called upon them. She feels socially isolated. She has a 4-year college degree.

Mrs. J reports a long history of intermittent periods of depression. She has done counseling in the past and feels she has "ok" coping skills. She has no history of suicidal ideation. She shares that she tends to become more "depressed" when she feels she has no control over her health and wellness. She is "tired of taking so many medications that don't even work."

Data Analysis

Basic descriptive frequencies were used to analyze demographic characteristics of the members of each group. Due to a small sample size in each group as well as ordinal data on the measure of self-efficacy, nonparametric tests for significance were utilized to identify any significant differences between and within the groups on measures of weight, systolic blood pressure, diastolic blood pressure, and self-efficacy at baseline and after the intervention.

Mann-Whitney U (MWU) tests for independent samples were used to identify significant differences between groups at baseline and postintervention. Then, for each group, Wilcoxon signed-rank tests were used to check for significant differences between pre- and postmeasures of weight, systolic blood pressure, diastolic blood pressure, and self-efficacy within the group. The significance level was set at $\alpha = 0.05$, and all tests were conducted using a two-tailed test for significance. The small sample size prohibited any tests using covariates.

Project Outcome

The intervention group demonstrated improved systolic blood pressure readings postintervention in contrast to the comparison group. Additionally, there was significant improvement in systolic blood pressure from preintervention to postintervention within the intervention group. Although there was no significant change demonstrated in weight between the groups, the average weight loss in the intervention group was 4 pounds. The MWU tests revealed significant differences between the two groups in systolic blood pressure at the postintervention measurement time point (MWU = 167.5, p = .001). There were no other significant group differences in pre- and postintervention measures of diastolic blood pressure and weight, nor were there baseline group differences in systolic blood pressure (Table 11.2).

The Wilcoxon signed-rank test revealed significant differences between pre- and post-systolic blood pressure measures in the intervention group (Wilcoxon T = -3.186, p = .001). The number of negative differences was 13, indicating that 13 participants in the intervention group had a lower postintervention systolic blood pressure compared to preintervention blood pressure. There were no significant differences between pre- and postintervention diastolic blood pressure in this group. Significant differences in weight were found in the intervention group (Wilcoxon T = -2.232, p = .026), an average of 4 pounds per participant between pre- and postmeasures of weight (Table 11.3).

Self-efficacy scores increased in both groups, with a more significant improvement in the intervention group. The Wilcoxon signed-rank test was used to identify any significant changes in pre- to postintervention self-efficacy scores, and each group was analyzed separately. There was a significant difference in pre- and post–self-efficacy scores for both groups (Table 11.4).

TABLE 11.2 *Independent Mann-Whitney* U *Test Pre- and Postintervention Measures Comparing Groups*

	Intervention Group ($n = 14$) Mean Rank	Comparison Group ($n = 14$) Mean Rank
Systolic blood pressure preintervention	15.25	13.75
Systolic blood pressure postintervention*	9.54	19.46
Diastolic blood pressure preintervention	13.14	15.86
Diastolic blood pressure postintervention	12.07	16.93
Weight preintervention	13.79	15.21
Weight postintervention	13.54	15.46

* MWU = 167.5, p = .001.

TABLE 11.3 *Wilcoxon Signed-Rank Scores Blood Pressure and Weight T1–T2*

	Intervention Group (n = 14) Standard Test Statistic	p value	Comparison Group (n = 14) Standard Test Statistic	p value
Systolic blood pressure	−3.186	.001	−.346	.729
Diastolic blood pressure	−1.517	.129	−1.381	.167
Weight	−2.232	.026	−.237	.812

TABLE 11.4 *Self-Efficacy Mean Scores*

	Intervention Group	Comparison Group	Mann-Whitney U
Self-efficacy T1	9.18	19.82	172.5; $p < .001$
Self-efficacy T2	11.46	17.54	140.5; $p < .025$
Wilcoxon signed-rank scores T1–T2	3.081	2.871*	

*$p < .001$.

These findings are consistent with other studies of group visits. Additional support group visits help to enhance confidence among patients in their self-care management (Davis, Sawyer, & Vinci, 2008; Jaber et al., 2006b; Jaber, Braksmajer, & Trilling, 2006c; Masley, Phillips, & Copeland, 2000; Sadur et al., 1999; Scott et al., 2004; Trento et al., 2004; Watts et al., 2009; Yehle, Sands, Rhynders, & Newton, 2009).

The improvements found in systolic blood pressure and self-efficacy in the study group may well be related to the increased visit time allotted to the intervention group in contrast with the comparison group. The longer visit time allows for a comprehensive review of guidelines; education on the importance of screening and follow-up care; medication management; and preventive approaches including nutrition, exercise, and stress management. The group visit program also promotes goal setting at the end of each visit and review of goals at the start of each subsequent visit. The group visit format provides a venue for patients to learn from and support each other, enhancing confidence in self-care management.

CASE STUDY PART II

Mrs. J Participates in the Intervention

Mrs. J was seen in the office by the NP three times, each visit lasting 30 to 45 minutes. A comprehensive health review was completed and reviewed with Mrs. J. The review helped to evaluate genetic, environmental, and lifestyle risk factors impacting Mrs. J's health and

(continued)

(continued)

wellness. Motivational interviewing was used as the foundational intervention during the individual visits. She started in a contemplative stage of change in which she was able to verbalize her physical and behavioral health issues and was beginning to feel ready to start working on them. During the third visit Mrs. J moved from a contemplative stage of change to an action stage, at which time she opted to enroll in the hypertension group visit 12-week program.

Throughout the 12-week course of the program the groups met four times formally with the NP, and the group itself organized a daily walking group 5 days per week. With the guidance of the NP and the support of her coworkers also enrolled in the group visit program, Mrs. J was very committed to making steady lifestyle modifications. Mrs. J was able to arm herself with the knowledge to goal set and successfully carry them out. With each goal that Mrs. J set and reached she verbalized her increased self-confidence. Mrs. J was able to make healthy changes in her diet and started participating in the group's walking group. She shared that her energy level was on the rise and her depressive symptoms were decreasing each day. Eight weeks into the program Mrs. J's fasting glucose levels were significantly lower and her blood pressure was so low that we took her off of her amlodipine. By the end of the 12-week group visit program we had cut her lisinopril to half the dose she had been on when she started the program, and her systolic and diastolic blood pressure was in control. Mrs. J had also lost 10 pounds. Her self-efficacy scores went from 9 to15.

Preprogram Biometrics Screening	Postprogram Biometrics Screening
BMI: 58.7	BMI: 56.7
Weight: 350 lbs	Weight: 340 lbs
Waist circumference: 51	Waist circumference: 50
BP: 164/98	BP: 128/80
Blood glucose: 160	Blood glucose: 128
Hb-A1c: 7.2	Hb-A1c: 6.1
Total cholesterol: 250	Total cholesterol: 230
HDL: 38	HDL: 37
LDL: 160	LDL: 128
Triglycerides: 247	Triglycerides: 220
Preprogram Self-Efficacy	**Postprogram Self-Efficacy**
9	15

BMI, body mass index; BP, blood pressure; Hb-A1c, hemoglobin A1C; HDL, high-density lipoprotein; LDL, low-density lipoprotein.

Outcome

Almost 1 year post program, Mrs. J continues to have once-a-month health coaching visits. She has lost 67 pounds and walks 1 mile per day. She is no longer on citalopram to control her depression, as she feels she has been empowered and educated to use healthier non-pharmacological coping skills.

IMPACT

This capstone project demonstrated patient outcomes related to better control of systolic blood pressure and weight among the group visit participants. It also showed an increase in self-efficacy among participants in both the intervention and the comparison groups. The project, conducted in a natural clinic setting, demonstrated the viability of group visits for improving health parameters among patients with hypertension. A limitation of this capstone is that the results cannot be generalized. This project was nonrandomized, did not control for length of visits, had small numbers, and did not control for type or amount of medications.

Although the sample size was small, the findings were statistically significant and at minimum provide validation for further investigation. Further studies using larger sample sizes are warranted in line with national health goals to improve fiscal responsibility in health care, demonstrate positive patient outcomes, and enhance both patient and provider satisfaction.

REFERENCES

Abramowitz, S. A., Flattery, D., Franses, K., & Berry, L. (2010). Linking a motivational interviewing curriculum to the chronic care model. *Journal of General Internal Medicine, 25*(Suppl. 4), 620–626. doi:10.1007/s11606-010-1426-6

Centers for Disease Control and Prevention. (2011, February 4). Vital signs: Prevalence, treatment, and control of hypertension—United States, 1999–2002 and 2005–2008. *Morbidity and Mortality Weekly Report, 60*(4), 103–108.

Davis, A. M., Sawyer, D. R., & Vinci, L. M. (2008). The potential of group visits in diabetes care. *Clinical Diabetes, 26*(2), 58–62. doi:10.2337/diaclin.26.2.58

Davis, K. (2012). *Expenditures for hypertension among adults age 18 and older, 2009: Estimates for the U.S. civilian noninstitutionalized population* (Statistical Brief No. 371). Retrieved from http://www.meps.ahrq.gov/mepsweb/data_files/publications/st371/stat371.shtml

Edelman, D., Fredrickson, S. K., Melnyk, S. D., Coffman, C. J., Jeffreys, A. S., Datta, S., . . . Weinberger, M. (2010). Medical clinics versus usual care for patients with both diabetes and hypertension: A randomized trial. *Annals of Internal Medicine, 152*(11), 689–696. doi:10.7326/0003-4819-152-11-201006010-00001

Houck, S., Kilo, C., & Scott, J. C. (2003). Improving patient care: Group visits 101. *Family Practice Management, 10*(5), 66–68.

Jaber, R., Braksmajer, A., & Trilling, J. (2006a). Group visits: A qualitative review of current research. *Journal of the American Board of Family Medicine, 19*(3), 276–290. doi:10.3122/jabfm.19.3.276

Jaber, R., Braksmajer, A., & Trilling, J. (2006b). Group visits for chronic illness care: Models, benefits and challenges. *Family Practice Management, 13*(1), 37–40.

Jaber, R., Braksmajer, A., & Trilling, J. (2006c). Group visits: Our experience with this adjunctive model to chronic care management. *Internet Journal of Family Practice, 4*(1).

Masley, S., Phillips, S., & Copeland, J. R. (2001). Group office visits change dietary habits of patients with coronary artery disease: The dietary intervention and evaluation trial (DIET). *Journal of Family Practice, 50*(3), 235–239.

Mohammadi, E., Abedi, H. A., Gofranipour, F., & Jalali, F. (2002). Partnership caring: A theory of high blood pressure control in Iranian hypertensives. *International Journal of Nursing Practice, 8*(6), 324–329. doi:10.1046/j.1440-172X.2002.00386.x

Ong, K. L., Cheung, B. M., Man, Y. B., Lau, C. P., & Lam, K. S. (2007). Prevalence, awareness, treatment, and control of hypertension among United States adults 1999–2004. *Hypertension, 49*(1), 69–75. doi:10.1161/01.HYP.0000252676.46043.18

Ostby, T., Yarnall, K. S., Krause, K. M., Pollak, K. I., Gradison, M., & Michener, J. L. (2005). Is there time for management of patients with chronic disease in primary care? *Annals of Family Medicine, 3*, 209–214.

Sadur, C. N., Moline, N., Costa, M., Michalik, D., Mendolowitz, D., Roller, S., . . . Javorski, W. C. (1999). Diabetes management in a health maintenance organization. Efficacy of care management using cluster visits. *Diabetes Care, 22*(12), 2011–2017. doi:10.2337/diacare.22.12.2011

Schappert, S. M., & Rechtsteiner, E. A. (2011). Ambulatory medical care utilization estimates for 2007. *Vital Health Statistics. Series 13, Data from the National Health Survey,* (169), 1–38. Retrieved from http://www.cdc.gov/nchs/data/series/sr_13/sr13_169.pdf

Scott, J. C., Conner, D. A., Venohr, I., Gade, G., McKenzie, M., Kramer, A. M., . . . Beck, A. (2004). Effectiveness of a group outpatient visit model for chronically ill older health maintenance organization members: A 2-year randomized trial of cooperative health care clinic. *Journal of the American Geriatrics Society, 52*(9), 1463–1470. doi:10.1111/j.1532-5415.2004.52408.x

Sheridan, S., Pignone, M., & Donahue, K. (2003). Screening for high blood pressure: Review of the evidence for the U.S. Preventive Services Task Force. *American Journal of Preventive Medicine, 25*(2), 151–158. doi:10.1016/S0749-3797(03)00121-1

Stanford Patient Education Center, Stanford School of Medicine. (2014). *Self-Efficacy for Managing Chronic Disease 6-Item Scale.* Retrieved from http://patienteducation.stanford.edu/research/secd6.html

Trento, M., Passera, P., Borgo, E., Tomalino, M., Bajardi, M., Cavallo, F., & Porta, M. (2004). A 5-year randomized controlled study of learning, problem solving ability, and quality of life modifications in people with type 2 diabetes managed by group care. *Diabetes Care, 27*(3), 670–675. doi:10.2337/diacare.27.3.670

United States Department of Health & Human Services. (2004). *The seventh report of the Joint National Committee on Prevention, Detection, Evaluation and Treatment of High Blood Pressure.* Washington, DC: U.S. Government Printing Office. Retrieved from https://www.nhlbi.nih.gov/guidelines/hypertension

Wagner, E. H., Austin, B. T., Davis, C., Hindmarsh, M., Schaefer, J., & Bonomi, A. (2001). Improving chronic illness care: Translating evidence into action. *Health Affairs, 20*(6), 64–78. doi:10.1377/hlthaff.20.6.64

Wang, Y., & Wang, Q. J. (2004).The prevalence of prehypertension and hypertension among US adults according to the new Joint National Committee guidelines: New challenges of the old problem. *Archives of Internal Medicine, 164*(19), 2126–2134. doi:10.1001/archinte.164.19.2126

Watts, S. A., Gee, J., O'Day, M. E., Schaub, K., Lawrence, R., Aron, D., & Kirsh, S. (2009). Nurse practitioner-led multidisciplinary teams to improve chronic illness care: The unique strengths of nurse practitioners applied to shared medical appointments/group visits. *Journal of the American Academy of Nurse Practitioners, 21*(3), 167–172. doi:10.1111/j.1745-7599.2008.00379.x

Yehle, K. S., Sands. L. P., Rhynders, P. A., & Newton, G. D. (2009). The effect of shared medical visits on knowledge and self-care in patients with heart failure: A comparison study. *Heart & Lung, 38*(1), 25–33. doi:10.1016/j.hrtlng.2008.04.004

Yoon, S. S., Burt, V., Louis, T., & Carroll, M. D. (2012). *Hypertension among adults in the United States, 2009–2010* (NCHS Data Brief, No. 107). Hyattsville, MD: National Center for Health Statistics. Retrieved from http://www.cdc.gov/nchs/data/databriefs/db107.htm

12

The Clinical Case Narrative: Preparing the DNP Nurse to Deliver Comprehensive Care

Janice Smolowitz and Judy Honig

DNP Essential #8

Advanced practice nursing

American Association of Colleges of Nursing. (2006). *The essentials of doctoral education for advanced nursing practice.* Retrieved from http://www.aacn.nche.edu/publications/position/DNPEssentials.pdf

This chapter describes the DNP portfolio as the capstone project for clinical DNP programs.

It exemplifies DNP *Essential #8* as it relates to development of competency-based benchmarks and assessment measures of clinical scholarship reflective of advanced practice nursing.

Barbara A. Anderson, Editor

FOCUS

The focus of the Columbia University School of Nursing (CUSON) clinical doctorate is to prepare graduates to provide comprehensive, evidence-based care to a panel of patients over time and across clinical settings. The DNP portfolio, tailored to fit with the focus of the program, is the capstone project submitted in partial fulfillment of the DNP degree. The CUSON DNP portfolio represents the culminating project that demonstrates the attainment, application, and synthesis of knowledge of doctoral-level advanced nursing practice. It is the compilation of accomplishment accrued by the DNP student during learning experiences and activities in coursework and practica, and in particular, during the integrative final practicum, the DNP residency.

The portfolio as the capstone project for clinical DNP programs is described. The portfolio is a competency-based, comprehensive benchmark and assessment measure of clinical scholarship for DNP students whose focus is the provision of comprehensive cross-site clinical care for individuals and populations. Components of the DNP portfolio are identified and explained in detail. In addition, the link between the DNP competencies and the final DNP portfolio capstone are presented.

REVIEW OF THE LITERATURE

A portfolio is a tangible record of student accomplishments and provides documentation for competency-based assessment of complex clinical performance. Portfolios have been used in the education of health care professionals to promote learning by actively engaging the student to bridge theory and practice; to foster reflective practice; and to measure, assess, and appraise clinical performance, professionalism, and clinical scholarship (Butani, Blankenburg, & Long, 2013; Byrne, Schroeter, Carter, & Mower, 2009; McMullan et al., 2003; Wittmann-Price, 2012). Portfolios offer a robust format as a formative and summative assessment in the health professions and provide the foundation for future life-long learning and scholarship.

The national recommendation for DNP education as described in *The Essentials of Doctoral Education for Advanced Nursing Practice* (American Association of Colleges of Nursing [AACN], 2006) states that all programs include a final integrative practice immersion experience that provides the context for the final DNP project. As described by the AACN (2006), the final project should demonstrate the synthesis of knowledge attainment and practice expertise. The final project should demonstrate mastery of an advanced practice specialty. In a clinical program, this expertise focuses on patient care. Demonstration of mastery for an advanced practice specialty, as described in the DNP *Essentials*, is as follows:

- Use of evidence to improve practice or patient outcomes
- Tangible and deliverable academic product
- Documentation of outcome of the DNP student's educational experience
- Measurable outcome to evaluate the immersion experience
- Summary of the student's growth in knowledge and expertise
- Provides the foundation for future scholarly practice (AACN, 2006, p. 20)

THE DNP PORTFOLIO

In alignment with the AACN recommendation, the CUSON DNP portfolio is a measurable and scholarly outcome, generated during the final practicum, in which students present the application of knowledge and evidence into practice.

In the portfolio, using the *DNP Competencies of Comprehensive Care* (CUSON, 2011) as the guide, the student demonstrates a strong interaction between the final project and the integrative practicum. DNP graduates describe this synergistic experience as transformational. This reflective process fosters professional growth and is an approach to lifelong learning and scholarship. Based on the relevancy for clinicians and advanced practice nursing, the DNP Portfolio can be viewed as the preferred format for the final project for DNP programs that focus on the provision of direct care to a patient population.

Documentation of Competency-Based DNP Education

The CUSON *DNP Competencies in Comprehensive Care* (2011) forms the framework for the curriculum, is integrated throughout the coursework and practicums, and provides the structure for the portfolio. These competencies are divided into four domains: (1) Comprehensive Clinical Care, (2) Interdisciplinary and Patient-Centered Communication, (3) Systems and Context of Care, and (4) Building and Using Evidence for Best Clinical Practice. The competencies are further described by performance objectives, which are measurable behaviors that can be assessed through student documentation, observation, and reflective classroom discussion (see Table 12.1).

TABLE 12.1 *DNP Competencies in Comprehensive Care and Performance Objectives for Direct Comprehensive Patient Care 2011*

DNP students specializing in comprehensive care will demonstrate expertise in the provision, coordination, and direction of comprehensive care to patients, including those who present in healthy states and those who present with complex, chronic, and/or comorbid conditions, across clinical sites and over time. The DNP student will:

Domain (D) 1. Comprehensive Clinical Care	
Competency (C) 1	**Performance Objective (PO)**
Evaluate patient needs based on genetic profile, family history, age, developmental stage, and individual risk to formulate plans for health promotion and disease prevention.	A. Identify a potential genetic risk.
	B. Diagnose a genetic condition.
	C. Evaluate individual patient needs based on age, developmental stage, family history, ethnicity, and individual risk.
	D. Formulate a plan that addresses health promotion, anticipatory guidance, and/or disease prevention for the individual.
	E. Develop a plan that addresses health promotion, anticipatory guidance, and/or disease prevention for the family.

(continued)

TABLE 12.1 *DNP Competencies in Comprehensive Care and Performance Objectives for Direct Comprehensive Patient Care 2011 (continued)*

Competency (C) 2

Evaluate health risk utilizing principles of epidemiology and clinical prevention.

Performance Objective (PO)

A. Assess the patient/family at risk for a condition, incorporating epidemiological principles and/or environmental factors that contribute to risk/incidence of disease.

B. Assess the patient/family *with* a condition, incorporating epidemiological principles and/or environmental factors that contribute to risk/incidence of disease.

Competency (C) 3

Formulate differential diagnoses, diagnostic strategies, and therapeutic interventions with attention to scientific evidence, safety, and cost for patients who present with new conditions and those with ambiguous or incomplete data, complex illnesses, and comorbid conditions.

Performance Objective (PO)

A. Formulate a differential diagnosis for a patient who presents with new, undifferentiated signs and symptoms.

B. Formulate a differential diagnosis for a patient who presents with ambiguous or incomplete data, complex illnesses, comorbid conditions, and potential multiple diagnoses.

C. Discuss the rationale for the differential diagnosis.

D. Discuss the rationale for the diagnostic evaluation with attention to scientific evidence, safety, cost, invasiveness, simplicity, acceptability, adherence, and efficacy.

E. Discuss the rationale for the therapeutic intervention with attention to scientific evidence, safety, cost, invasiveness, simplicity, acceptability, adherence, and efficacy.

Competency (C) 4

Appraise acuity of patient condition, determine need to transfer patient to higher-acuity setting, coordinate and manage transfer to optimize patient outcomes.

Performance Objective (PO)

A. Assess the acuity of patient status.

B. Determine the most appropriate treatment setting based on level of acuity.

C. Formulate a transfer plan.

D. Implement plan to transfer the patient to a higher level of care utilizing written and oral communication.

E. Coordinate care during transition to the higher-acuity setting.

F. Comanage care in person, or

G. Comanage care though written and verbal instructions.

H. Recommendations for patient disposition from the higher-acuity location.

I. Coordination of postdischarge care.

(continued)

TABLE 12.1 *DNP Competencies in Comprehensive Care and Performance Objectives for Direct Comprehensive Patient Care 2011 (continued)*

Competency (C) 5	Performance Objective (PO)
Evaluate and direct care during hospitalization, and design a comprehensive discharge plan for patients from an acute care setting.	A. Assess the acuity of patient's condition and determine the most appropriate inpatient treatment setting based on level of acuity. B. Actively participate in the admission process to the appropriate inpatient treatment setting. C. Actively comanage patient care during hospitalization. D. Formulate plan for ongoing care to be provided in a subacute setting, such as a long-term care facility, rehabilitation facility, or home or community setting. E. Coordinate ongoing comprehensive care to be provided in a subacute setting, such as a long-term care facility, rehabilitation facility, or home or community setting.
Competency (C) 6	**Performance Objective**
Direct comprehensive care for patient in a subacute setting to maximize quality of life and functional status.	A. Assess the acuity of the patient's condition to determine the need for subacute, long-term care. B. Determine the most appropriate subacute or chronic care treatment setting based on level of acuity, functional status, and availability of formal and informal caregiver resources. C. Coordinate ongoing comprehensive care provided in a subacute setting. D. Initiate referral to other health care professionals while maintaining primary responsibility for patient care in a subacute setting. E. Utilize consultant recommendations for decision making while maintaining primary responsibility for care in a subacute setting.

Domain (D) 2. Interdisciplinary and Patient-Centered Communication

Competency (C) 1	Performance Objective (PO)
Assemble a collaborative, Interdisciplinary network and refer and consult appropriately while maintaining primary responsibility for comprehensive patient care.	A. Initiate referral to other health care professionals while maintaining primary responsibility for patient care. B. Accept referrals from other health care professions and communicate consultation findings and recommendations to the referring provider and collaborative network. C. Utilize consultation recommendations for decision making while maintaining primary responsibility for care.

(continued)

TABLE 12.1 *DNP Competencies in Comprehensive Care and Performance Objectives for Direct Comprehensive Patient Care 2011 (continued)*

	D. Evaluate outcomes of interventions.
	E. Provide ongoing patient follow-up and monitor outcomes of collaborative network interventions.
Competency (C) 2 Coordinate and manage the care of patients with chronic illness, utilizing specialists, other disciplines, community resources, and family, while maintaining primary responsibility for direction of patient care as the focus of care transitions across ambulatory to acute, subacute, and community settings.	**Performance Objective (PO)** A. Coordinate care for a patient with chronic illness as the focus of care transitions across ambulatory, acute, subacute, and/or community settings. B. Comanage care for a patient with chronic illness as the focus of care transitions across ambulatory, acute, subacute, and/or community settings. C. Coordinate care for a patient with chronic illness utilizing specialists, other disciplines, community resources, and family. D. Direct care for patient with chronic illness and ensure the seamless flow of information among providers as the focus of care transitions across settings. E. Comanage care for a patient with chronic illness utilizing shared decision making and teaching. F. Comanage care for a patient with chronic pain as the focus of care transitions across ambulatory, acute, subacute, and/or community settings.
Competency (C) 3 Translate health information, incorporating shared decision making and addressing the specific needs of a patient in the context of family and community.	**Performance Objective (PO)** A. Assess and tailor health information for the individual patient's needs. B. Promote shared decision making with patient and caregivers. C. Apply the principles of health literacy in interactions with the patient.
Competency (C) 4 Facilitate and guide the process of palliative care and/or planning end-of-life care and promote informed choices and shared decision making by patient, family, and members of the health care team.	**Performance Objective (PO)** A. Facilitate and guide the palliative care process by discussing diagnoses and prognoses, clarifying and validating patient desires and priorities, and promoting informed choices and shared decision making by the patient, family, and members of the health care team. B. Facilitate and guide planning of end-of-life care by discussing diagnoses and prognoses, clarifying and validating patient desires and priorities, and promoting informed choices and shared decision making by the patient, family, and members of the health care team.

(continued)

TABLE 12.1 *DNP Competencies in Comprehensive Care and Performance Objectives for Direct Comprehensive Patient Care 2011 (continued)*

Domain (D) 3. Systems and Context of Care	
Competency (C) 1 Construct and evaluate outcomes of a culturally sensitive, individualized intervention.	**Performance Objective (PO)** A. Assess culturally specific needs of the patient in the context of family and community. B. Construct a culturally sensitive intervention to address the needs of the patient in the context of family and community. C. Evaluate outcomes of the intervention. D. Tailor health information to the patient and caregiver's cultural needs. E. Provide effective individualized health care.
Competency (C) 2 Evaluate gaps in health care access that compromise optimal patient outcomes and apply current knowledge of the organization and financing of health care systems to advocate for the patient and to ameliorate negative impact.	**Performance Objective (PO)** A. Identify gaps in access that compromise the patient's optimum care. B. Identify gaps in reimbursement that compromise the patient's optimum care. C. Demonstrate patient advocacy in the provision of continuous and comprehensive care. D. Apply current knowledge of the organization to ameliorate negative impact. E. Apply current knowledge of health care systems to ameliorate negative impact.
Competency (C) 3 Synthesize the principles of legal and ethical decision making and analyze dilemmas that arise in patient care, interprofessional relationships, research, or practice management to improve outcomes.	**Performance Objective (PO)** A. Synthesize ethical principles to address a complex practice dilemma. B. Apply ethical principles to resolve the dilemma. C. Synthesize legal principles to address a complex practice dilemma. D. Apply legal principles to resolve the dilemma.
Competency (C) 4 Integrate principles of business, finance, economics, and/or health policy to design an initiative that benefits a group of patients, practice, community, and/or a population.	**Performance Objective (PO)** A. Identify barriers to quality, cost, and/or access to care. B. Develop practice initiatives to address quality, cost, or access to effective care. C. Implement and guide practice and/or system change that incorporates principles of business, finance, economics, and/or health policy. D. Evaluate outcomes of practice initiative.

(continued)

TABLE 12.1 *DNP Competencies in Comprehensive Care and Performance Objectives for Direct Comprehensive Patient Care 2011 (continued)*

Domain (D) 4. Building and Using Evidence for Best Clinical Practices and Scholarship

Competency (C) 1
Synthesize and analyze evidence from practice, clinical information systems, and patient databases using reflection, interpretation, and cumulative clinical knowledge.

Competency (C) 2
Evaluate quality of care against standards using reliable and valid methods and measures and propose innovative, interdisciplinary models that enhance outcomes.

Competency (C) 3
Critically appraise and synthesize research findings and other evidence to inform practice and policy for optimal patient outcomes.

Competency (C) 4
Assess and critically appraise clinical scholarship through participation in the peer review process.

Competency (C) 5
Utilize informatics tools to build data to identify best practices and to identify deficits and improve delivery of care.

The DNP Competencies in Comprehensive Care are compatible with *The Essentials of Doctoral Education for Advanced Nursing Practice* (2006) and the National Organization of Nurse Practitioner Faculties (NONPF) Core Nurse Practitioner Competencies (2012). In particular, because of the focus on comprehensive clinical care, the CUSON DNP competencies provide more depth and breadth in *Essential VIII, Advanced Nursing Practice*. The relationship among the CUSON, AACN (2006), and NONPF (NONPF, 2012) competencies are described in Table 12.2.

TABLE 12.2 *Comparison of the CUSON DNP Competencies in Comprehensive Care, the AACN Essentials of Doctoral Education for Advanced Nursing Practice, and the NONPF Nurse Practitioner Core Competencies*

CUSON DNP Competencies in Comprehensive Care (2011)	AACN Essentials of Doctoral Education for Advanced Nursing Practice (2006)	NONPF Nurse Practitioner Core Competencies (2012)
DNP students specializing in comprehensive care will demonstrate expertise in the provision, coordination, and direction of comprehensive care to patients, including those who present in healthy states and those who present with complex, chronic, and/or comorbid conditions across clinical sites and over time. The DNP student will:	The following DNP *Essentials* outline the curricular elements and competencies that must be present in programs conferring the Doctor of nursing practice degree. The DNP *Essentials* delineated here address the foundational competencies that are core to all advanced nursing practice roles.	Scientific Foundation Leadership Quality Practice Inquiry Technology & Information Literacy Health Delivery System Ethical Competencies Independent Practice
Domain 1. Comprehensive Clinical Care		
Competency 1: Evaluate patient needs based on genetic profile, family history, age, developmental stage, and individual risk to formulate plans for health promotion and disease prevention.	*Essential I*: Scientific Underpinnings for Practice *Essential VII*: Clinical Prevention and Population Health for Improving the Nation's Health *Essential VIII*: Advanced Nursing Practice	Scientific Foundation Quality Practice Inquiry Health Delivery System Independent Practice

(continued)

TABLE 12.2 *Comparison of the CUSON DNP Competencies in Comprehensive Care, the AACN Essentials of Doctoral Education for Advanced Nursing Practice, and the NONPF Nurse Practitioner Core Competencies (continued)*

CUSON DNP Competencies in Comprehensive Care (2011)	AACN Essentials of Doctoral Education for Advanced Nursing Practice (2006)	NONPF Nurse Practitioner Core Competencies (2012)
Competency 2: Evaluate health risk utilizing principles of epidemiology and clinical prevention.	*Essential II*: Organizational and Systems Leadership for Quality Improvement and Systems Thinking *Essential VII*: Clinical Prevention and Population Health for Improving the Nation's Health *Essential VIII*: Advanced Nursing Practice	Scientific Foundation Quality Practice Inquiry Independent Practice
Competency 3: Formulate differential diagnoses, diagnostic strategies, and therapeutic interventions with attention to scientific evidence, safety, and cost for patients who present with new conditions and those with ambiguous or incomplete data, complex illnesses, and comorbid conditions.	*Essential III*: Clinical Scholarship and Analytical Methods for Evidence-Based Practice *Essential VIII*: Advanced Nursing Practice	Health Delivery System Quality Independent Practice
Competency 4: Appraise acuity of patient condition, determine need to transfer patient to higher-acuity setting, coordinate and manage transfer to optimize patient outcomes.	*Essential VI*: Interprofessional Collaboration for Improving Patient and Population Health Outcomes *Essential VIII*: Advanced Nursing Practice	Health Delivery System Quality Independent Practice

(continued)

TABLE 12.2 *Comparison of the CUSON DNP Competencies in Comprehensive Care, the AACN Essentials of Doctoral Education for Advanced Nursing Practice, and the NONPF Nurse Practitioner Core Competencies (continued)*

CUSON DNP Competencies in Comprehensive Care (2011)	AACN Essentials of Doctoral Education for Advanced Nursing Practice (2006)	NONPF Nurse Practitioner Core Competencies (2012)
Competency 5: Evaluate and direct care during hospitalization and design a comprehensive discharge plan for patients from an acute care setting.	*Essential VI*: Interprofessional Collaboration for Improving Patient and Population Health Outcomes *Essential VIII*: Advanced Nursing Practice	Health Delivery System Quality Independent Practice
Competency 6: Direct comprehensive care for patients in a subacute setting to maximize quality of life and functional status.	*Essential VI*: Interprofessional Collaboration for Improving Patient and Population Health Outcomes *Essential VIII*: Advanced Nursing Practice	Health Delivery System Quality Independent Practice
Domain 2. Interdisciplinary and Patient-Centered Communication		
Competency 1: Assemble a collaborative interdisciplinary network, refer and consult appropriately while maintaining primary responsibility for comprehensive patient care.	*Essential II*: Organizational and Systems Leadership for Quality Improvement and Systems Thinking *Essential VI*: Interprofessional Collaboration for Improving Patient and Population Health Outcomes *Essential VIII*: Advanced Nursing Practice	Health Delivery System Quality Independent Practice

(*continued*)

TABLE 12.2 *Comparison of the CUSON DNP Competencies in Comprehensive Care, the AACN Essentials of Doctoral Education for Advanced Nursing Practice, and the NONPF Nurse Practitioner Core Competencies (continued)*

CUSON DNP Competencies in Comprehensive Care (2011)	AACN Essentials of Doctoral Education for Advanced Nursing Practice (2006)	NONPF Nurse Practitioner Core Competencies (2012)
Competency 2: Coordinate and manage the care of patients with chronic illness utilizing specialists, other disciplines, community resources, and family, while maintaining primary responsibility for direction of patient care as the focus of care transitions across ambulatory to acute, subacute, and community settings.	*Essential II*: Organizational and Systems Leadership for Quality Improvement and Systems Thinking *Essential VI*: Interprofessional Collaboration for Improving Patient and Population Health Outcomes *Essential VIII*: Advanced Nursing Practice	Health Delivery System Quality Independent Practice
Competency 3: Translate health information, incorporating shared decision making and address the specific needs of a patient in context of family and community.	*Essential II*: Organizational and Systems Leadership for Quality Improvement and Systems Thinking *Essential III*: Clinical Scholarship and Analytical Methods for Evidence-Based Practice *Essential VIII*: Advanced Nursing Practice	Scientific Foundation Health Delivery System Quality Independent Practice
Competency 4: Facilitate and guide the process of palliative care and/or planning end-of-life care and promote informed choices and shared decision making by patient, family, and members of the health care team.	*Essential I*: Scientific Underpinnings for Practice *Essential III*: Clinical Scholarship and Analytical Methods for Evidence-Based Practice *Essential VIII*: Advanced Nursing Practice	Scientific Foundation Health Delivery System Independent Practice

(continued)

TABLE 12.2 *Comparison of the CUSON DNP Competencies in Comprehensive Care, the AACN Essentials of Doctoral Education for Advanced Nursing Practice, and the NONPF Nurse Practitioner Core Competencies (continued)*

CUSON DNP Competencies in Comprehensive Care (2011)	AACN Essentials of Doctoral Education for Advanced Nursing Practice (2006)	NONPF Nurse Practitioner Core Competencies (2012)
Domain 3. Sytems and Context of Care		
Competency 1: Construct and evaluate outcomes of a culturally sensitive, individualized intervention.	*Essential II*: Organizational and Systems Leadership for Quality Improvement and Systems Thinking *Essential III*: Clinical Scholarship and Analytical Methods for Evidence-Based Practice *Essential VIII*: Advanced Nursing Practice	Scientific Foundation Quality Independent Practice
Competency 2: Evaluate gaps in health care access that compromise optimal patient outcomes, and apply current knowledge of the organization and financing of health care systems to advocate for the patient and to ameliorate negative impact.	*Essential II*: Organizational and Systems Leadership for Quality Improvement and Systems Thinking *Essential V*: Health Care Policy for Advocacy in Health Care *Essential VIII*: Advanced Nursing Practice	Policy Quality Leadership Independent Practice
Competency 3: Synthesize the principles of legal and ethical decision making and analyze dilemmas that arise in patient care, interprofessional relationships, research, or practice management to improve outcomes.	*Essential I*: Scientific Underpinnings for Practice *Essential VIII*: Advanced Nursing Practice	Scientific Foundation Ethical Competencies Independent Practice

(continued)

TABLE 12.2 *Comparison of the CUSON DNP Competencies in Comprehensive Care, the AACN Essentials of Doctoral Education for Advanced Nursing Practice, and the NONPF Nurse Practitioner Core Competencies (continued)*

CUSON DNP Competencies in Comprehensive Care (2011)	AACN Essentials of Doctoral Education for Advanced Nursing Practice (2006)	NONPF Nurse Practitioner Core Competencies (2012)
Competency 4: Integrate principles of business, finance, economics, and/ or health policy to design an initiative that benefits a group of patients, practice, community, and/or a population.	*Essential II*: Organizational and Systems Leadership for Quality Improvement and Systems Thinking *Essential V*: Health Care Policy for Advocacy in Health Care	Policy Quality Leadership
Domain 4. Building and Using Evidence for Best Clinical Practices and Scholarship		
Competency 1: Synthesize and analyze evidence from practice, clinical information systems, and patient databases using reflection, interpretation, and cumulative clinical knowledge.	*Essential III*: Clinical Scholarship and Analytical Methods for Evidence-Based Practice *Essential VIII*: Advanced Nursing Practice	Scientific Foundation Quality Practice Inquiry Independent Practice
Competency 2: Evaluate quality of care against standards using reliable and valid methods and measures and propose innovative, interdisciplinary models that enhance outcomes.	*Essential III*: Clinical Scholarship and Analytical Methods for Evidence-Based Practice *Essential V*: Health Care Policy for Advocacy in Health Care	Policy Quality Practice Inquiry
Competency 3: Critically appraise and synthesize research findings and other evidence to inform practice and policy for optimal patient outcomes.	*Essential I*: Scientific Underpinnings for Practice *Essential III*: Clinical Scholarship and Analytical Methods for Evidence-Based Practice *Essential V*: Health Care Policy for Advocacy in Health Care *Essential VIII*: Advanced Nursing Practice	Scientific Foundation Policy Quality Practice Inquiry Independent Practice

(continued)

TABLE 12.2 *Comparison of the CUSON DNP Competencies in Comprehensive Care, the AACN Essentials of Doctoral Education for Advanced Nursing Practice, and the NONPF Nurse Practitioner Core Competencies (continued)*

CUSON DNP Competencies in Comprehensive Care (2011)	AACN Essentials of Doctoral Education for Advanced Nursing Practice (2006)	NONPF Nurse Practitioner Core Competencies (2012)
Competency 4: Assess and critically appraise clinical scholarship through participation in the peer review process.	*Essential III*: Clinical Scholarship and Analytical Methods for Evidence-Based Practice *Essential VI*: Interprofessional Collaboration for Improving Patient and Population Health Outcomes	Scientific Foundation Independent Practice
Competency 5: Utilize informatics tools to build data to identify best practices and to identify deficits and improve delivery of care.	*Essential III*: Clinical Scholarship and Analytical Methods for Evidence-Based Practice *Essential IV*: Information Systems/Technology and Patient Care Technology for the Improvement and Transformation of Health Care *Essential VIII*: Advanced Nursing Practice	Scientific Foundation Technology & Information Literacy Health Delivery System

AACN, American Association of Colleges of Nursing; CUSON, Columbia University School of Nursing; DNP, Doctor of Nursing Practice; NONPF, National Organization of Nurse Practitioner Faculties.

Consistent with the national recommendations, the crucial educational component of the DNP program is the residency, an academic, mentored, integrative clinical experience in which the student assimilates and synthesizes knowledge and achieves the doctoral competencies in the provision of comprehensive patient care. The student demonstrates assimilation of knowledge and the translation of knowledge into practice in the DNP portfolio. The DNP portfolio is a structured self-reflection and self-analysis of the student's practice. It is a quantitative and qualitative document and includes multiple competency-based assessment measures. The components of the portfolio demonstrate the attainment of scholarship, self-evaluation, and a plan for future continued learning.

The components of the DNP portfolio are:

A minimum of seven in-depth, evidence-based reflective clinical practice
   case narratives that provide evidence of competent, comprehensive
   practice
Primary authorship publication in a peer-reviewed journal
A group or individual project with a systems approach that benefits a
   group of patients, practice, community, and/or a population
A detailed summary of the clinical encounters and population demo-
   graphics that are representative of the integrative practicum
A plan for self-evaluation and continued learning
Curriculum vitae
Classroom, clinical teaching, and pedagogy
Additional peer-reviewed journal articles, peer-reviewed book chapters,
   and peer-reviewed presentations such as grand rounds

Table 12.3 displays how the components of the portfolio link to the
competencies.

Some examples of scholarly papers, reports, and publications are presented
in Table 12.4.

TABLE 12.3 *DNP Competencies in Comprehensive Care and the DNP Portfolio Component*

Competency	Portfolio Component
Domain 1. Comprehensive Clinical Care	
Competency 1 Evaluate patient needs based on genetic profile, family history, age, developmental stage, and individual risk to formulate plans for health promotion and disease prevention.	Portfolio Case Narrative Academic Papers, Reports, and Presentations High-Risk Genomics Case Study
Competency 2 Evaluate health risk utilizing principles of epidemiology and clinical prevention.	Portfolio Case Narrative Academic Papers, Reports, and Presentations Epidemiology Paper
Competency 3 Formulate differential diagnoses, diagnostic strategies, and therapeutic interventions with attention to scientific evidence, safety, and cost, for patients who present with new conditions and those with ambiguous or incomplete data, complex illnesses, and comorbid conditions.	Portfolio Case Narrative

(continued)

TABLE 12.3 *DNP Competencies in Comprehensive Care and the DNP Portfolio Component (continued)*

Competency	Portfolio Component
Competency 4 Appraise acuity of patient condition, determine need to transfer patient to higher-acuity setting, coordinate and manage transfer to optimize patient outcomes.	Portfolio Case Narrative
Competency 5 Evaluate and direct care during hospitalization, and design a comprehensive discharge plan for patients from an acute care setting.	Portfolio Case Narrative
Competency 6 Direct comprehensive care for patient in a subacute setting to maximize quality of life and functional status.	Portfolio Case Narrative Academic Papers, Reports, and Presentations Chronic Illness Management Presentation
Domain 2. Interdisciplinary and Patient-Centered Communication	
Competency 1 Assemble a collaborative interdisciplinary network, refer and consult appropriately while maintaining primary responsibility for comprehensive patient care.	Portfolio Case Narrative
Competency 2 Coordinate and manage the care of patients with chronic illness utilizing specialists, other disciplines, community resources, and family while maintaining primary responsibility for direction of patient care as the focus of care transitions across ambulatory to acute, subacute, and community settings.	Portfolio Case Narrative Academic Papers, Reports, and Presentations Interdisciplinary Committee Membership
Competency 3 Translate health information, incorporating shared decision making, and address the specific needs of a patient in the context of family and community.	Portfolio Case Narrative Academic Papers, Reports, and Presentations
Competency 4 Facilitate and guide the process of palliative care and/or planning end-of-life care and promote informed choices and shared decision making by the patient, family, and members of the health care team.	Portfolio Case Narrative Academic Papers, Reports, and Presentations

(continued)

TABLE 12.3 *DNP Competencies in Comprehensive Care and the DNP Portfolio Component (continued)*

Competency	Portfolio Component
Domain 3. Systems and Context of Care	
Competency 1 Construct and evaluate outcomes of a culturally sensitive, individualized intervention.	Portfolio Case Narrative
Competency 2 Evaluate gaps in health care access that compromise optimal patient outcomes and apply current knowledge of the organization and financing of health care systems to advocate for the patient and to ameliorate negative impact.	Portfolio Case Narrative Academic Papers, Reports, and Presentations Chronic Illness Systems Change Presentation
Competency 3 Synthesize the principles of legal and ethical decision making and analyze dilemmas that arise in patient care, interprofessional relationships, research, or practice management to improve outcomes.	Portfolio Case Narrative Academic Papers, Reports, and Presentations Ethics Paper
Competency 4 Integrate principles of business, finance, economics, and/or health policy to design an initiative that benefits a group of patients, practice, community, and/or a population.	Systems Project Academic Papers, Reports, and Presentations Practice Management Project
Domain 4. Building and Using Evidence for Best Clinical Practices and Scholarship	
Competency	Portfolio Component
Competency 1 Synthesize and analyze evidence from practice, clinical information systems, and patient databases using reflection, interpretation, and cumulative clinical knowledge.	Systems Project Manuscripts and Publications Academic Papers, Reports, and Presentations Systematic Review/Meta-Analysis Paper Summary of electronic log using graphics from program to profile your patient population
Competency 2 Evaluate quality of care against standards using reliable and valid methods and measures and propose innovative, interdisciplinary models that enhance outcomes.	Manuscripts and Publications Systems Project Academic Papers, Reports, and Presentations

(continued)

TABLE 12.3 *DNP Competencies in Comprehensive Care and the DNP Portfolio Component (continued)*

Competency	Portfolio Component
Competency 3 Critically appraise and synthesize research findings and other evidence to inform practice and policy for optimal patient outcomes.	Manuscripts and Publications Systems Project Academic Papers, Reports, and Presentations Policy, Legislation, and/or Regulatory Issue Paper
Competency 4 Assess and critically appraise clinical scholarship through participation in the peer-review process.	Manuscripts and Publications Academic Papers, Reports, and Presentations Policy, Legislation, and/or Regulatory Issue Paper Goal Statement
Competency 5 Utilize informatics tools to build data to identify best practices and to identify deficits and improve delivery of care.	Systems Project Academic Papers, Reports, and Presentations Informatics Paper and Presentation

TABLE 12.4 *Examples of DNP Students' Scholarly Papers, Presentations, and Individual and Group Projects*

Systematic Reviews

Angú, L., Velloria, E., Envaina, E., & Malone, A. (2012). Mediastinitis and blood transfusion in cardiac surgery: A systematic review. *Heart & Lung, 41*(3), 255–263. doi:10.1016/j.hrtlng.2011.07.012

Domeny, M. (in press). Vitamin D: The great debate. *Clinical Scholars Review.*

Kramps, M., Flanagan, A., & Smaldone, A. (2013). The use of vitamin K supplementation to achieve INR stability: A systematic review and meta-analysis. *Journal of the American Association of Nurse Practitioners, 25*(10), 535–544. doi:10.1111/1745-7599.12022

Massingham, K., Fox, S., & Smaldone, A. (2013). Asthma therapy in pediatric patients: A systematic review of treatment with montelukast versus inhaled corticosteroids. *Journal of Pediatric Health Care.* Advance online publication. doi:10.1016/j.pedhc.2012.11.005

Systematic Approach to Care

Madden, R., Kane, H., & Eisner, R. (2013). Obesity self-management education: A community-based project for an underserved population. *Clinical Scholars Review, 6*(1), 30–38. doi:http://dx.doi.org/10.1891/1939-2095.6.1.30

(continued)

TABLE 12.4 *Examples of DNP Students' Scholarly Papers, Presentations, and Individual and Group Projects (continued)*

Roedel, F. D. (in press). Telenutrition: An integrated approach to delivering medical nutrition therapy to bariatric surgery patients via synchronous tele-consultation. *Clinical Scholars Review.*

Ethical Issues

Corsaro, M. (2011). Patient requested induction of labor: Examining an ethical dilemma. *Online Journal of Health Ethics, 7*(1), 1–9.

McCreary, K. E. (2012). Elder abuse: Ethical decision making. *Clinical Scholars Review, 5*(1), 55–59. doi:http://dx.doi.org/10.1891/1939-2095.5.1.55

Ulysse, F. G., Balicas, M., & Xu, Y. (2011). Ethical dilemma: Therapeutic nondisclosure. *Clinical Scholars Review, 4*(2), 115–118. doi:http://dx.doi.org/10.1891/1939-2095.4.2.115

Case Studies

Blanton, K. (2011). Female genital cutting and the health care provider's dilemma: A case study. *Clinical Scholars Review, 4*(2), 119–124. doi:http://dx.doi.org/10.1891/1939-2095.4.2.119

Lamarca, N. H., Golden, L., John, R. M., Naini, A., De Vivo, D. C., & Sproule, D. M. (2012). Diabetic ketoacidosis in an adult patient with spinal muscular atrophy type II: Further evidence of extraneural pathology due to survival motor neuron 1 mutation? *Journal of Child Neurology, 28*(11), 1517–1520. doi:10.1177/0883073812460096

Peters, M. M. (in press). The use of anti-retroviral therapy in the prevention of HIV transmission among serodiscordant couples. *Clinical Scholars Review.*

Veloria, E. (in press). Lambl's excrescence: An uncommon cause of cardioembolic stroke. *Clinical Scholars Review.*

Wuhrman, E., & Clark, M. (2011). Use of ephedrine for the short-term treatment of postoperative nausea and vomiting: A case report. *Journal of Perianesthesia Nursing, 26*(5), 305–309. doi:10.1016/j.jopan.2011.06.003

Podium and Poster Presentations

McEneany, M., Corsaro, M., Evangeslista, M. C., & Holuba, N. (2011, March). *A systematic review of treatment approaches for adolescents with polycystic ovary syndrome.* Poster presented at the meeting of Eastern Nursing Research Society 23rd Annual Scientific Sessions, Philadelphia, PA.

Massingham, K., & Fox, S. (2012, March). *Asthma therapy in pediatric patients: A systematic review of montelukast versus inhaled corticosteroids.* Poster presentation at the meeting of Eastern Nursing Research Society 24th Annual Scientific Sessions, New Haven, CT.

LaMarca, N. (2011, June). *Congenital heart disease and spinal muscular atrophy.* Presented at meeting of International Spinal Muscular Atrophy Research Group 15th Annual Meeting, Orlando, FL.

Roszel, E., & More, S. (2013, April). *The association between eating disorders and substance use in youth and young adults: A systematic review and meta-analysis.* Poster presentation at the meeting of Eastern Nursing Research Society 25th Annual Scientific Sessions, Boston, MA.

Demonstrating the Scholarship of Comprehensive Care

The most prominent feature of the DNP portfolio is the evidence-based, reflective, detailed clinical case narrative. The case narrative format was developed to provide a framework for students to systematically document clinical encounters and for faculty to evaluate performance (Smolowitz & Honig, 2008). The narrative's descriptive quality provides a basis for understanding the complex cognitive processes, in-depth reflection, high-level analysis and synthesis, and critical appraisal and application of evidence required for the provision of clinical care. Case narratives may depict a single encounter or complex management over time and across settings. Through case narrative writing, students demonstrate competence in the provision and coordination of direct care for patients, including those who present in healthy states and those who present with complex, chronic, and/or co-morbid conditions, across clinical settings and over time.

Clinical case narrative writing is integrated into the curriculum. Throughout the course of study, students engage in clinical field experiences and clinical seminars. Clinical case narrative writing is taught in the clinical seminar to promote the scholarship of practice, integration of evidence-based practice, and peer evaluation of clinical decision making. Analysis of real-life scenarios provides students with insight into their own decision-making processes in the context of the realities and challenges of actual clinical practice.

During clinical seminars, students write, present, and critically appraise each other's narratives, which are based on patient interactions during the concurrent field experience. This activity reinforces the educational material presented in research and evidence-based practice courses as well as practice management, genomics, epidemiology, and chronic illness management. Students are constantly being challenged to apply theoretical and research data presented in class to real life situations. Discussion of decision making and possible alternative choices based on reading establishes and reinforces the process of life-long learning and the scholarship of practice.

The scholarly process of case narrative writing continues into the residency. Case narratives for the portfolio are compiled during the residency. During the residency, each student is assigned a clinical mentor who facilitates clinical opportunities so that the student can meet the competencies of comprehensive care. Each student is also assigned a residency advisor who guides the case narrative writing process. While working with their advisors, students post their case narratives in the online course room discussion board to request peer feedback regarding the entire narrative or a specific question. Writing the narrative is an interactive process that may include mentor, peer, and advisor feedback.

When the advisor determines that the competencies of the narrative have been met, the case narrative is sent to the residency director. The residency director assigns the case to a DNP portfolio narrative reader for review and comment. The DNP narrative readers have preparation in the same clinical specialty as the DNP resident. Graduates of the program often choose to serve as case narrative readers to continue to participate in the scholarship of practice. The case narrative reader reviews the case for utilization of proper format, content, utilization of evidence, and determines if the competency is addressed.

The reader may offer suggestions for improvement. This constructive critique is returned to the advisor who informs the student. The case is reviewed and the suggestions are addressed.

This process continues until the case narrative is approved. If questions arise regarding the content of a specific narrative, the residency director independently reviews the narrative with other experts and provides a decision. When all the components of the portfolio have been attained, including approval of all case narratives and agreement that all direct care competencies have been met, the student submits the completed portfolio for review by the portfolio committee. The portfolio committee reviews and approves the portfolio and makes a recommendation that the DNP degree be granted.

Case Narrative Format

All narratives include the care provided, assessments supported by evidence, outcomes of the interventions, as well as the specific CUSON DNP direct care competencies and performance objectives.

Documentation of Domain

Competencies and performance objectives within the narrative: Performance objectives of a competency are met by behaviors that direct the outcome of the case narrative. The student documents actions that demonstrate competency and performance objectives to explicate education, counseling, treatment interventions, referrals, consultations, or clinical decision making.

Example of Demonstrating the Achievement of a Competency

A referral to the nearby epilepsy center is scheduled. The soonest appointment is available in 2 months. I explain the urgent need for the evaluation but the scheduling personnel explains there are no sooner appointments and there is nothing she can do. I call a neurologist who specializes in epilepsy and review the case and request assistance with this referral. The neurologist agrees with my assessment and will assist (Domain [D]2, Competency [C]1, Performance Objective [PO]A).

The reader is able to review this section and determine if the student has met the criteria for Domain 2, Competency 1, and Performance Objective A. The general goal of this competency is to assemble a collaborative interdisciplinary network, and refer and consult appropriately while maintaining primary responsibility for comprehensive patient care. The specific performance objective or action that the student states she has documented in this section is performance objective A: Initiate referral to other health care professionals while maintaining primary responsibility for patient care. The portfolio reader who reviewed this case agreed that the student's actions specifically addressed performance objective A in this section (see Table 12.1, presenting performance objectives linked with competencies).

The case narrative is based on clinical encounter patient notes. Patient data is de identified according to Health Insurance Portability and Accountability Act (HIPAA) guidelines when the narrative is written. When choosing a patient care scenario to write as a narrative, the student is advised to "write to the competency." Essentially, the student tells the story of the care provided so the reader can assess if the care is consistent with current standards and the competency is met as determined by achievement of specific performance objectives. The key sections of the narrative are described below.

Introduction to the Case Narrative

Each case narrative begins with a paragraph that discusses the reason for selecting the case, total number of encounters in the narrative, clinical settings (ambulatory, home, acute, emergency department, medical floor in an acute care hospital, skilled nursing facility, rehabilitation center), type of insurance (commercial, Medicaid, Medicare, self-pay), and the competency or competencies addressed in the case study. The introduction is the only section written in the past tense.

Example of the Introduction

This case describes the care I provided for a 60-year-old Hispanic male with Medicare insurance who had metastatic esophageal cancer. This case narrative focuses on four office appointments surrounding pain management and palliative care over a period of 3 weeks. The case narrative addresses the following CUSON doctoral competency for direct patient care.

Domain 2, Competency 1

Assemble a collaborative interdisciplinary network; refer and consult appropriately while maintaining primary responsibility for comprehensive patient care.

> PO A. Initiate referral to other health care professionals while maintaining primary responsibility for patient care
>
> PO B. Accept referrals from other health care professions and communicate consultation findings and recommendations to the referring provider and collaborative network
>
> PO C. Utilize consultation recommendations for decision making while maintaining primary responsibility for care
>
> PO D. Evaluate outcomes of interventions

Summary of Care Provided Prior to Case Narrative

This section is only included when the student assumes care for a patient known to a practice or addresses care prior to the time period that is the focus of the case narrative. Information not specific to the competency is presented in summary form. This provides the reader with background information about the patient while focusing attention on the competency addressed within the body of the narrative. The summary of care includes each of the following points for problems that will be active during the provision of care: initial diagnosis (time of diagnosis), relevant clinical findings, diagnostic tests, interventions, patient response to most recent therapeutic intervention, and proposed plan.

Example of Summary of Care

The patient is a 4-year-old female who is an established patient in the practice. She has come to this practice since she was born. Last year she was referred to early intervention. The one evaluation took 6 months to complete. She was diagnosed with pervasive developmental disorder – not otherwise specified (PDD-NOS) 6 months ago by a developmental specialist.

Encounter Context

The case narrative begins with the encounter context, which provides information to orient the reader to the initial encounter with regard to setting, time, context, patient demographics, and DNP role.

Example of Encounter Context

Encounter 1: Initial evaluation
DNP role: I am an adult nurse practitioner and DNP resident seeing this patient for initial consult visit.
Identifying information:
    Site: Urban academic medical center
    Setting: Cardiology specialty private office practice
    Reason for encounter: Initial evaluation, referral note on prescription pad from community physician.
    Informant: Patient and wife, who state the doctor heard a murmur, did a test, and sent us to you. The referral note from the community physician states "92-year-old man with newly diagnosed severe aortic stenosis, please evaluate and treat." No other medical records are available.

Patient Encounter or Encounters

The student's deidentified notes form the basis for this section. Some narratives begin with an initial comprehensive patient encounter, whereas other narratives begin with a follow-up encounter, which builds from the summary of care. All encounters are written in the present tense. Most encounters will include some or all of the following information: chief complaint in patient's own words or other source if patient is nonresponsive; history of present illness; active medical problems being treated that are not related to presenting complaint; past health history, social history, and family history, which includes genogram; review of systems (not related to chief complaint, physical examination, laboratory data review, outside medical record review, impression, and plan; Smolowitz, Honig, & Reinisch, 2010).

For each new or undifferentiated problem identified, the student writes a paragraph that describes the possible diagnoses from most to least likely, based upon the patient's history, pertinent positive and negative physical examination findings, diagnostic tests, and risk factors. The student discusses the probability for each diagnosis and provides a rationale for selecting the most likely diagnosis, which forms the basis of the plan. In situations where there is a potentially life-threatening diagnosis that must be excluded before other diagnoses can be entertained, the student provides a rationale for decision making and how the plan will proceed once this diagnosis is excluded or confirmed. When previously identified acute or self-limiting health care issues resolve, they are documented in the impression and plan of care. At appropriate intervals, the plan of care may also address ongoing health problems, health maintenance, and immunizations according to established guidelines.

Citing and Leveling the Evidence

After appropriate sections of the case narrative, in italics, the scientific underpinnings or the evidence for clinical decision making are cited. This evidence has usually been published within the past 5 years. Sources of evidence include primary sources, meta-analysis, or expert guidelines. The level of evidence for each source is cited using the University of Oxford Center for Evidence-Based Medicine (CEBM) guidelines (CEBM, 2009).

Example of Impression With Evidence Citation

The patient is a 4-year-old Caucasian female who presents with her mother for a routine well-child examination and to discuss difficulty with sleep. The patient was recently diagnosed with pervasive developmental disorder – not otherwise specified (PDD-NOS) and autism spectrum disorder (ASD). There are safety concerns during the night due to her sleep disturbance.

Differential diagnoses for difficulty with sleep in a child include abnormal sleep/wake cycle or abnormal circadian rhythm, behavioral insomnia, bedtime fears, difficulty with limit setting, obstructive sleep apnea, and narcolepsy. An abnormal sleep/wake cycle is the most likely diagnosis. Children with ASD are thought to have decreased levels of the hormone melatonin and often have difficulty sleeping. Melatonin is a hormone that helps regulate the sleep/wake cycle.

Melatonin levels typically increase when it is dark outside and decrease when it gets light out. Previous research has shown that children with ASD have a higher prevalence of sleep abnormalities than typically developing children, with a prevalence from 40% to 85%. This is thought to be due to decreased levels of physiologic melatonin and/or abnormal melatonin circadian rhythms. Children present with longer sleep-onset latency, frequent awakening during the night, and reduced sleep duration (Rossignol & Frye, 2011).

CEBM, level 1

Critical Appraisal

When appropriate to a section of the case narrative, a detailed discussion of the DNP student's thought processes is included as a critical appraisal section in a box. The critical appraisal may be particularly important to an ethical discussion or when there is conflicting or ambiguous evidence. The critical appraisal may not necessarily appear in all or any of a student's case narratives. However, faculty have noted that as students begin to provide cross-site care for persons with complex comorbid conditions and there is no evidence specific to a diagnosis, the utilization of the critical appraisal becomes increasingly important. In the clinical setting, the student has limited time and resources when making a decision. Writing the case narrative and including a critical appraisal afford the opportunity to explore the literature and decision-making process with the mentor, advisor, and peers. The critical appraisal box allows the student to step out of the case context and discuss alternative options for addressing a specific clinical dilemma.

APPENDIX

The appendix includes information that is relevant to the case but too detailed to include in the body of the narrative as it would distract from competency focus. Appendices can include DSM criteria, validated assessment tools, and institution-specific policies and protocols. The first appendix includes all medications discussed in the case narrative and briefly identifies salient indications, pharmacokinetics, and contraindications that are specific to the patient.

The Portfolio of the Future: The DNP With Focus in Comprehensive Care

The portfolio, as currently conceived, provides students an opportunity to demonstrate clinical competency and scholarship in the provision of comprehensive cross-site clinical care for individuals and populations in the context of the *DNP Competencies in Comprehensive Care* (2011), *AACN Essentials* (2006), and *NONPF Competencies* (2012). While the portfolio is used to profile students' accomplishments, it also serves as a source for individual reflection.

Graduates from the CUSON program report intermittently reviewing their portfolios. The graduates consider the short- and long-term goals they developed prior to graduation in light of the trajectory of career choices. Graduates continue to value the insights, dedication, and colleagueship required to write clinical case narratives. Some students have commented that the evidence used to support clinical decisions at the time the case was written has subsequently changed. The standard of care no longer requires such extensive diagnostic testing. Former students question if the outcome of the case would have differed if current standards were applied. Graduates also consider the cost of care and how societal demands have changed the settings in which this type of care is now delivered. Graduates who are now educators in Master's and DNP programs report using the narratives and the format as a teaching strategy. Others have adapted the format and apply the case narrative writing process for use with systems projects.

As the role of the DNP prepared to deliver comprehensive care evolves, the portfolios of future students will also evolve so that these portfolios will reflect advances in scholarship, clinical practice, education, technology, and individual growth. The portfolio of the future should be electronic and designed to reflect accomplishments as the DNP student transitions to the professional role and assumes new responsibilities in a variety of settings.

The e-portfolio provides a mechanism by which students can highlight and modify content to reflect new achievements. While the current portfolio focuses on written work, the digital portfolio will utilize audio, video, and graphics to illustrate accomplishments. It will be portable and link to supplemental information, which supports the stated position. The portfolio of the future has the potential to more accurately depict the individual strengths and professional development of each DNP student. The e-portfolio has the potential to be an enduring professional dossier and a repository of ongoing accomplishments. As such, it may become integrated into the certification and certification-maintenance processes.

Certification is a mechanism for assuring the public that direct care providers have met the minimum requirements for providing care within a specific focus. The DNP-prepared nurse in comprehensive care has the opportunity to take the American Board of Comprehensive Care (ABCC) examination and be credentialed as a diplomate of comprehensive care (ABCC, 2012). The purpose of this examination is to test graduates' knowledge of the clinical science considered essential for the sophisticated practice of comprehensive care. The examination emphasizes evaluating severity of patient problems, managing therapy, and using clinical judgment among mainstream illnesses. While ambulatory patient encounters are emphasized, inpatient encounters of significant complexity are also represented. This examination may be included in the portfolio of the future (ABCC, 2012).

The DNP nurse with focus in comprehensive clinical care is prepared to treat individuals in the context of family and community, across settings and transitions, and over time. The DNP nurse is also involved in evaluating care for a population of patients and developing context-specific interventions. The portfolio as an evolving document provides the opportunity for demonstrating participation in these activities. The portfolio, which began as a student capstone project, can demonstrate growth and achievement throughout the individual's career. As we move into the future and seek to understand the totality of DNP graduates' contribution to health care, each section of the portfolio can be examined to better understand the contributions of these health care professionals.

REFERENCES

American Association of Colleges of Nursing. (2006). *The essentials of doctoral education for advanced nursing practice.* Retrieved from http://www.aacn.nche.edu/ publications/position/DNPEssentials.pdf

American Board of Comprehensive Care. (2012*). Mission and goal statement.* Retrieved from http://www.cumc.columbia.edu/nursing/dnpcert/abccmission.shtml

Byrne, M., Schroeter, K., Carter, S., & Mower, J. (2009). The professional portfolio: An evidence-based assessment method. *Journal of Continuing Education in Nursing, 40*(12), 545–552. doi:10.3928/00220124-20091119-07

Butani, L., Blankenburg, R., & Long, M. (2013). Stimulating reflective practice among your learners. *Pediatrics, 131*(2), 204–206. doi:10.1542/peds.2012-3106

Columbia University School of Nursing. (2011). *DNP competencies for comprehensive care.* Retrieved from http://www.cumc.columbia.edu/nursing/academics/pdf/DNPCompetencies2011%282%29.pdf

McMullan, M., Endacott, R., Gray, M. A., Jasper, M., Miller, C. M., Scholes, J., & Webb, C. (2003). Portfolios and assessment of competence: A review of the literature. *Journal of Advanced Nursing, 41*(3), 283–294. doi:10.1046/j.1365-2648.2003.02528.x

National Organization of Nurse Practitioner Faculties. (2012). *Nurse practitioner core competencies.* Retrieved from https://c.ymcdn.com/sites/nonpf.siteym.com/resource/resmgr/competencies/npcorecompetenciesfinal2012.pdf

Rossignol, D. A., & Frye R. E. (2011). Melatonin in autism spectrum disorders: A systematic review and meta-analysis. *Developmental Medicine and Child Neurology, 53*(9), 783–792. doi:10.1111/j.1469-8749.2011.03980.x

Smolowitz, J., & Honig, J. (2008). DNP portfolio: The scholarly project for doctor of nursing practice. *Clinical Scholars Review, 1*(1), 18–22. doi:http://dx.doi.org/10.1891/1939-2095.1.1.18

Smolowitz, J., Honig J., & Reinisch, C. (Eds.). (2010). *Writing DNP clinical case narratives: Demonstrating and evaluating competency in comprehensive care.* New York, NY: Springer Publishing Company.

University of Oxford, Centre for Evidence Based Medicine. (2009, March). *Levels of evidence.* Retrieved from http://www.cebm.net/index.aspx?o= 1025

Wittmann-Price, R. A. (2011). *Fast facts for developing a nursing academic portfolio: What you need to know in a nutshell.* New York, NY: Springer Publishing Company.

The DNP Capstone: Influencing Clinical Outcome

Get to the table and be a player, or someone who does not understand nursing will do that for you.

—Loretta Ford

13

The Impact of DNP Projects on Quality and Safety in Health Care Organizations

Carol Patton

Major issues confronting the U.S. health care system include the increasing burden of chronic diseases; finite capacity to deliver safe, reliable, economic, and just health care; and poorly coordinated interprofessional care that is culturally relevant, patient centered, and cost effective (Fisher, 2011). There will be an escalation in demand for health care services in the next decade, with an aging population requiring increased health care services (McLaughlin & Kaluzny, 2005). The increase in demand for services comes at a time when the U.S. government is trying to curb health care spending on chronic disease care. While there are concerns with regard to level of insurance coverage, the more compelling challenges are quality and safety.

Patient quality and safety has become a looming issue. The government, particularly the Centers for Medicare and Medicaid Services (CMS), has made quality and safety a national health care priority. As a result, health care organizations now use the measures outlined in the Health Care Employer Data and Information Sets (HEDIS) to assess performance on quality of care. These HEDIS performance measures reflect patient perception of health care experience (Eddy et al., 2008).

Health care organizations that survive in the 21st century are going to be those that create and sustain an organizational mission and philosophy of quality and safety. Health care organizations must embrace values, focusing on care that ensures every patient receives the right care, in the right way, in every health care encounter. *Value-driven* health care is focused on health outcome achieved for the resources invested (Sollecito & Johnson, 2013). While value-driven care is imperative, many health care organizations are operated as business models

(Walston & Chou, 2012). Organizational strategic plans focus on quality- and safety-driven outcomes with emphasis on cost. Nurses, with all levels of nursing education, have experienced the complexity and challenges between business aspects of the organization and providing quality care while working in health care organizations (Wilson, Whitaker, & Whitford, 2012).

The Role of DNP Projects in Patient Safety and Quality Outcomes

This health care environment provides numerous opportunities for doctor of nursing practice (DNP) projects to examine gaps between desired and actual patient safety and quality outcomes. Further, there is a compelling need for DNP students to embrace the health care business model and to examine strategies that allow them to practice to the full extent and scope of practice as described in *The Future of Nursing: Leading Change, Advancing Health* (Institute of Medicine, 2010).

DNP projects can provide compelling learning opportunities to support health care organizations in their mission to create cultures of value-driven care, especially around support of quality and safety initiatives. Linking the DNP project to value-driven care that enhances quality and safety is based on three specific elements: the mission and philosophy of the health care organization; the structure and function of the health care organization; and the predetermined clinical outcomes related to patient safety and quality. Table 13.1 indicates the characteristics of these three specific elements guiding the DNP project.

DNP students have numerous opportunities to partner with a variety of health care organizations to examine historical as well as contemporary aggregate data reflecting on systems issues. For example, the DNP project might examine aggregate organizational data and metrics on time and flow in the post-anesthesia recovery room (PAR). There are numerous key stakeholders involved in patient flow through the PAR, including but not limited to surgeons, nurses, patient care technicians, operating room staff, emergency room staff, emergency surgery patients, families, floors awaiting patient return or admission from the PAR, and business managers concerned about staffing and overtime. Flow can impact many key stakeholders. A DNP project might examine best practices and examine models of care that inform and expedite patient safety and quality of the patient encounter in the PAR. Conversely, the project might focus on the cost–benefit ratio of a new staffing plan in the PAR based on a meta-analysis of relevant, contemporary literature.

Creating the Environment for a Successful DNP Project

Before initiating a DNP project, there are several key elements that must be in place in order to ensure a successful and positive DNP project experience. These elements include mentoring, time management, organizational and academic support, and planning for dissemination of the results. See Table 13.2 describing the key elements for successful DNP project development.

TABLE 13.1 *Elements Guiding the DNP Project*

Specific Elements	Rationale	Linkage of the Characteristic to a Final DNP Project
Driving mission and philosophy of the health care organization	The health care organization mission and philosophy indicate the values and strategic initiatives, including satisfaction of customers, constituency and key stakeholders, and performance measures	The DNP project analyzes and synthesizes aggregate data or metrics to determine gaps in patient safety and quality based on the health care organization mission and philosophy EXAMPLE: The infection rates for patients with catheter-associated urinary tract infections are exceeding ranges set by the CMS and this is impacting the health care reimbursement for the organization.
Structure and function of the health care organization	The structure and function of the organizations reflects the sincerity and due diligence in providing the highest level of value-driven service	The DNP project develops a microsystem change within the structure of the organization to enhance patient safety and outcomes EXAMPLE: The health care organization adds a state-of-the-art birthing suite with the latest amenities and technology to improve patient safety and quality as well as patient and staff satisfaction.
Predetermined, proactive patient quality and safety clinical outcomes	The health care organization focuses on best practices, integrating recognized clinical guidelines to provide exceptional quality of care and patient outcomes	The DNP project examines evidence and best practice to improve benchmarks and quality indicators for patient safety and quality EXAMPLE: Based upon meta analysis and synthesis of research literature, the DNP project identifies best practice leading to a policy change in care.

CMS, Centers for Medicare and Medicaid; DNP, doctor of nursing practice.

TABLE 13.2 *Key Elements for a Successful DNP Project*

Key Elements	Supporting Rationale
Mentor	The DNP student must have a mentor in the health care organization to navigate the system. While a doctoral degree is not essential, the mentor must be politically astute and offer guidance and support with resources within the health care system. EXAMPLE: The DNP student may be working with data or processes that are confidential and sensitive. The mentor can facilitate access to data and help problem solve when obstacles arise.
Timeline	The DNP student must have an adequate, realistic timeline and plan before beginning the project. EXAMPLE: Color-coded Gantt charts are a strategy for creating a timeline that is relevant and meaningful.
Organization Support	The DNP student must follow clinical guidelines and be familiar with the policies and processes within the organization. EXAMPLE: Health care organizations are responsible for any students entering their organization. The DNP students entering the facility must comply with regulations for immunizations and protection against infectious diseases.
Institutional Review Board Approval	The purpose of an IRB is to protect human subjects. Any time a DNP student is collecting data with plans to disseminate that data, there must be IRB approval. EXAMPLE: The health care organization may require internal organizational IRB approval in addition to the educational institution IRB approval process.
Timely Feedback	The DNP student requires timely content-focused feedback for the final DNP project. It is important to have adequate systems in place and a realistic timeline. EXAMPLE: It is unrealistic to submit a 30-page document to a faculty and expect a turnaround time on that document within 24 to 48 hours.
Disseminating Data	Expectations for the final deliverable and dissemination need to be built into the timeline. EXAMPLE: Failure to have an adequate timeline for disseminating data from the final DNP project, once again, may jeopardize program completion.

DNP, doctor of nursing practice; IRB, institutional review board.

Characteristics of Successful DNP Projects

The Essentials of Doctoral Education for Advanced Nursing Practice was developed by the DNP *Essentials* Task Force under the auspices of the American Association of Colleges of Nursing (AACN, 2006). The purpose of this document is to provide curricular and structural guidance for practice-focused doctoral education, including the DNP project (AACN, 2006). "Doctoral education, whether practice or research, is distinguished by completion of a specific project demonstrating synthesis of the students' work and laying the groundwork for future scholarship" (AACN, 2006, p. 20).

The thematic underpinning for all DNP projects should be a focus on application of scientific evidence to improve patient outcomes. The AACN does not prescribe the final deliverable for the final DNP project. There are multiple ways in which a DNP student could meet this deliverable. For example, the final DNP project could be a portfolio, linking components of the DNP practicum or course work with DNP *Essentials.* Or, it could be a document describing an evidence-based practice change at the clinical microsystem level. No matter what the DNP project is, it should be the foundation for future scholarly practice (AACN, 2006) and there must be a clear project goal and scope. The project goal then drives the methodology and strategy for the project, ensuring the final deliverable. Table 13.3 highlights examples of DNP project deliverables.

TABLE 13.3 *Examples of DNP Project Deliverables*

Project Deliverable	Example
Practice Change Initiative	A document that includes evidence of how a clinical practice change was planned, designed, implemented, and evaluated, including implications for practice and/or policy change in a clinical microsystem
Policy Change Within a Health Care Organization	A document that includes evidence of the process and outcomes used to examine evidence-based research and formulate an organizational change
Program Evaluation	An evaluation of the impact of a new program
Quality Improvement Project	A program that improves infection control on a postoperative surgical unit where multidose vials are being used for multiple patients
Evaluation of a New Practice Model	An examination of pre- and postintervention data on a new patient-centered care staffing model
Integrated Critical Literature Review	An in-depth review of previously published reports following rigorous methodological review guidelines on a clinical practice or policy issue

(continued)

TABLE 13.3 *Examples of DNP Project Deliverables (continued)*

Project Deliverable	Example
Meta Analysis	A meta-analysis reflecting examination of a large body of knowledge and providing a sophisticated synthesis of evidence (Russell, 2008, p. 241) The final deliverable consists of published and unpublished documents to inform evidence and analysis
Evidence-Based Clinical Practice Guideline	A document designed for clinical application based upon evidence-based clinical guidelines
Systematic Review of Literature	A thorough, comprehensive, scientifically rigorous, systematic review of literature that is systematic in formation of general questions being researched, searches for all relevant evidence on a clinical topic or issue, and summarizes the evidence The final deliverable would be a publishable document
Manuscript Submitted for Publication	A document submitted according to a predetermined peer-reviewed journal fulfilling editor guidelines and having a match with the mission and focus The manuscript is not an article until accepted for publication
Research Measurement Tool	A document to investigate valid and reliable tools for measuring a clinical concept This tool would involve a thorough review of research The final deliverable would be ready for publication
Executive Summary	A document summarizing a major practice change or executive decision supported by best practice and peer-reviewed data The final document would be prepared in executive summary format for presentation to a board of trustees in a health care organization

An excellent DNP project focus is an initiative to improve quality and safety within a health care organization. Consumers and health care organizations alike are focusing on value-driven health care that enhances quality and safety of care (Nelson, Batalden, Godfrey, & Lazar, 2011). The DNP student can research basic assumptions and rationale underlying value-driven care. See Table 13.4 for assumptions and rationale of value-driven care.

Health policy emerges from research studies, clinical practice guidelines, patient preference, and clinical data/process information from health care organizations (Grady, 2011). The DNP project can have policy implications and be a catalyst for sustainable change in these areas in health care organizations. Such

---

TABLE 13.4 *Assumptions and Rationale for Value-Driven Care Enhancing Quality and Safety*

Assumptions	Rationale
Health care to enhance patient safety and quality outcomes must be focused on culturally relevant self-care	Focusing on unique patient characteristics and needs enhances patient safety and quality outcomes Failure to focus on culturally relevant self-care, practices, and beliefs results in fragmented care that misses unique safety and quality issues
Plan of care must be patient centered	Health care organizations have largely operated on care of the system rather than value-driven, patient-centered care At present, health care organizations are evaluated and paid according to patient perception of the health care encounter
Decentralized health care systems are fragmented, presenting barriers to safety and quality outcomes	Health care organizations must strive to be suppliers of patient care at clinical microsystems levels (Patton, 2013)
Intra- and interprofessional health care teams support optimal patient safety and quality outcomes	High-reliability teams are comprised of intra- and interprofessional health care teams that focus on individual patients as the center of care (Patton, 2013)
Organizations that focus on patient quality and safety are moving to the forefront as high-reliability organizations	Reliability must focus on evaluation methods, calculation, and improvement of all operating performance in complex systems (Fisher, Bataldén, Godfrey, & Lazar, 2011)
Health care is a high-hazard industry	High-hazard organizations are prone to harm or kill There are often sentinel events or near misses as a result of the models of care currently used in U.S. health care delivery systems (Youngberg, 2011)
Quality and safety are interrelated guides to improvement	Quality and safety are science and must be examined from an evidence base Quality and safety grounded in evidence and best practice (Sherwood, 2012)

(continued)

TABLE 13.4 *Assumptions and Rationale for Value-Driven Care Enhancing Quality and Safety (continued)*

Assumptions	Rationale
Nurses, particularly DNP students, are in key roles to identify and influence patient quality and safety outcomes within health care organizations	Major areas with potential negative impact on patient quality and safety include: ■ The human factor ■ The system failure ■ Poor relationships and lack of communication between provider and patient ■ Failure to focus on a patient-centered plan of care ■ Inadequate staffing patterns and multitasking while performing critical tasks like medication administration ■ Root cause analysis of adverse events ■ Prioritizing and care coordination
Failure to focus on clinical microsystems results in errors in care that jeopardize quality and safety	The clinical microsystem in health care organizations provides excellent opportunity to assess and determine where, how, and why errors occur, including sentinel events and near-misses, impact on patient quality and safety (Nelson, Batalden, & Godfrey, 2007)

DNP, doctor of nursing practice.

TABLE 13.5 *Characteristics of Potential Clinical Microsystems for DNP Projects*

Characteristic	Description
Professional Nursing Identity	Moving from novice nurses to expert nurses using evidence-based clinical research integration
Nurse Vitality	Identifying the need for clinical practice or policy change to improve and enhance patient safety and quality outcomes
Clinical Practice Setting	Using a living clinical laboratory for determining effect and impact of practice change (Patton, 2013)
Clinical Microsystems for Patient Safety and Quality Issues	Relating safety, quality, and patient satisfaction issues to clinical microsystems, recognizing that health care organizations are held accountable for patient satisfaction and are reimbursed based upon meeting this criteria and value-based care
Outcomes at the Point of Care	Ensuring safety, quality, and patient satisfaction at the point of care The *point of care* is often referred to in literature as *The Sharp End of Care* The Sharp End of Care is "the point where the patient directly contacts the system" (Nelson et al., 2007, p. 74).

change can shape quality, safety, and patient-centered care. Supporting the development of a DNP project can be an excellent strategy for a health care organization fostering a health care culture that promotes, encourages, models, and incentivizes the translation of evidence into practice (Williams, 2012). DNP projects provide opportunity to examine micro-, macro-, or mesosystem levels linked to patient quality and safety issues. Focusing on health care at the microsystem level provides a new paradigm from which to examine clinical practice and create change, enhancing quality and safety outcomes. Table 13.5 provides examples of characteristics of potential clinical microsystems for DNP projects.

Nurses have always recognized clinical issues and sought to improve patient safety and outcomes (Nightingale, 1860/1946), and DNP projects now bring that recognition to a high level. DNP projects support health care organizations in the delivery of value-driven health care, especially around issues of patient safety and quality.

REFERENCES

American Association of Colleges of Nursing. (2006). *The essentials of doctoral education for advanced nursing practice*. Retrieved from www.aacn.nche.edu/publication/position/DNPEssentials.pdf

Eddy, D. M., Pawlson, L. G., Schaaf, D., Peskin, B., Shcheprov, A., Dziuba, J., . . . Eng, B. (2008). The potential effects of HEDIS performance measures on the quality of care. *Health Affairs, 27*(5), 1429–1441. doi:10.1377/hlthaff.27.5.1429

Fisher, E. (2011). Foreword. In E. C. Nelson, P. B. Batalden, M. M. Godfrey, & J. S. Lazar (Eds.), *Value by design: Developing clinical microsystems to achieve organizational excellence*. San Francisco, CA: Jossey-Bass.

Fisher, E. S., Batalden, P. B., Godfrey, M. M., & Lazar, J. S. (2011). *Value by design: Developing clinical microsystems to achieve organizational excellence*. San Francisco, CA: Jossey-Bass.

Grady, P. A. (2011). Research: A foundation for health policy. In A. S. Hinshaw & P. A. Grady (Eds.), *Shaping health policy through nursing research* (pp. 17–33). New York, NY: Springer Publishing Company.

Institute of Medicine. (2010). *The future of nursing: Leading change, advancing health*. Retrieved from http://www.iom.edu/~/media/Files/Report%20Files/2010/The-Future-of-Nursing/Future%20of%20Nursing%202010%20Recommendations.pdf

McLaughlin, C. P., & Kaluzny, A. D. (2005). Defining quality improvement: Past, present, and future. In C. P. McLaughlin & A. D. Kaluzny (Eds.), *Continuous quality improvement in health care: Theory, implications, and applications* (3rd ed., pp. 3–40). Sudbury, MA: Jones & Bartlett.

Nelson, E. C., Batalden, P. B., Godfrey, M. M., & Lazar, J. S. (Eds.). (2007). Foreword. In *Value by design: Developing clinical microsystems to achieve organizational excellence* (pp. xvii–xix). San Francisco, CA: Jossey-Bass.

Nightingale, F. (1946). *Notes on nursing: What it is, and what it is not*. Philadelphia, PA: J. B. Lippincott. Retrieved from https://archive.org/details/notesnursingwhat-00nigh. (Original work published 1860).

Patton, C. M. (2013, January). *Integration and application of high reliability theory by DNPs to enhance patient safety and quality.* Poster presented at meeting of the American Association of Colleges of Nursing, San Diego, CA.

Russell, C. L. (2008). Other sources of evidence. In N. A. Schmidt & J. M. Brown (Eds.), *Evidence-based practice for nurses: Appraisal and application of research* (pp. 235–249). Sudbury, MA: Jones & Bartlett.

Sherwood, G. (2012). Driving forces for quality and safety: Changing mindsets to improve health care. In G. Sherwood & J. Barnsteiner (Eds.), *Quality and safety in nursing: A competency approach to improving outcomes* (pp. 3–21). West Sussex, UK: John Wiley & Sons.

Sollecito, W. A., & Johnson, J. K. (2013). A call to action for transforming health care of the future. In W. A. Sollecito & J. K. Johnson (Eds.), *McLaughlon and Kaluzny's continuous quality improvement in health care* (4th ed., pp. 571–596). Burlington, MA: Jones & Bartlett.

Walston, S. L., & Chou, A. F. (2012). Strategic thinking and achieving competitive advantage. In L. R. Burns, E. H. Bradley, & B. J. Weiner (Eds.), *Shortell & Kaluzny's health care management: Organization, design and behavior* (6th ed., pp. 282–320). Clifton Park, NY: Delmar.

Williams, J. (2012). Creating a culture that promotes translation. In K. M. White & S. Dudley-Brown (Eds.), *Translation of evidence into nursing and health care practice* (pp. 175–190). New York, NY: Springer Publishing Company.

Wilson, A., Whitaker, N., & Whitford, D. (2012). Rising to the challenge of health care reform with entrepreneurial and intrapreneurial nursing initiatives. *Online Journal of Issues in Nursing, 17*(2), 5. Retrieved from http://nursingworld.org/MainMenuCategories/ANAMarketplace/ANAPeriodicals/OJIN/TableofContents/Vol-17-2012/No2-May-2012/Rising-to-the-Challenge-of-Reform.html

Youngberg, B. J. (2011). Creating systemic mindfulness: Anticipating, assessing, and reducing risks of health care. In B. J. Youngberg (Ed.), *Principles of risk management and patient safety* (pp. 293–303). Sudbury, MA: Jones & Bartlett.

14

Implementation and Dissemination of DNP Practice Scholarship

David G. O'Dell

How important is the actual implementation and dissemination of scholarly work performed by DNP graduates? A better question might be: If not implemented and disseminated, how many people will not benefit from improved health care outcome? Most would agree that there is value in the implementation and dissemination of scholarly work. The challenge is appreciating the themes, background, processes, and level of creativity that feeds into both implementation and dissemination.

This chapter will discuss definitions and concepts of dissemination, theoretical approaches to maximize dissemination, potential stakeholders, and opportunities for the nursing scholar. Performing doctoral scholarly work is admirable, but the work itself is not enough to truly demonstrate the potential of the doctoral practice degree. As the numbers of DNP graduates increase, the probability that health care outcomes will be impacted increases. However, this improvement can only take place with dissemination of experiences and knowledge.

DISSEMINATION: DEFINITIONS AND CONCEPTS

To disseminate is to scatter or diffuse a message. The word comes from Latin, meaning to sow from seed. The concept of dissemination implies the delivery of a product to customers, as in the world of advertising. The act of disseminating a message requires both a sender and a receiver, yet does not require feedback from the receiving audience. This can be seen in public announcements and speeches. Synonyms of dissemination are broadcast, spread, and propagate.

Does a product of scholarly work impact outcomes merely by being disseminated? If research findings and the application of these findings to practice are disseminated, will positive outcomes result? These are challenges for all disciplines striving to impact change.

THEORETICAL APPROACHES TO DISSEMINATION

The science of implementation and dissemination is evolving into a discipline that maximizes the skills of social sciences to deliver research and scientific findings to clinicians and practitioners. The Health Services Research Information Center (HSRIC), supported by the National Institutes of Medicine (IOM), disseminates information and associated evidence-based interventions (HSRIC, 2014). The National Institutes of Health (NIH) Office of Behavioral and Social Sciences Research (OBSSR) has funded research exploring implementation and dissemination of research findings (U.S. Department of Health and Human Services, NIH, OBSSR, 2013). OBSSR states that there is an enormous gap between knowledge and delivery:

> More present than ever within the research community is the belief that to optimize public health we must not only understand how to create the best interventions, but how to best ensure that they are effectively delivered within clinical and community practice. This is the focus of dissemination and implementation research, and building this knowledge base is imperative to get the best return on decades of investment in biomedical and behavioral research (2013, para.1).

According to Eagleman (2013), researchers have the following responsibilities in the public dissemination of scientific findings:

- Researchers owe understanding of knowledge generated to the people who fund the experiment, which may include the taxpaying public
- Research can leverage skills as scientists inspire critical thinking in public and political dialogue
- Researchers are optimally positioned to stem the flow of scientific misinformation in the media
- Researchers can explain the ways and means by which science can (and cannot) improve law and social policy
- Researchers must explain what science is and is not a way of thinking that upgrades our intuitions and requires tolerance of uncertainty
- The scientist is in the pleasurable position of being able to share the raw beauty of the world around us or inside of us. Scientists are optimally positioned to increase their presence in the public sphere, to synthesize large bodies of data, to weigh the evidence, and to communicate with nuance, sincerity, and exactitude.

While Eagleman (2013) addresses the social responsibility of researchers, the same expectations apply to professionals who translate evidence into practice. The expectation for the practice professional is perhaps more urgent compared to the researcher. Evidence-based practice can be implemented in multiple settings, replicated, and impact health care outcomes in ways appreciated by those outside of a select realm of practice. Researchers and practitioners must work collaboratively to inspire public dialogue and avoid misinformation by consumers.

Nursing researchers continue to deliver new knowledge on health care while the DNP-prepared professional translates and applies this knowledge to practice. Knowledge is translated into practice that improves health outcomes. Translation of evidence to practice has the potential of launching research findings into a level that the researcher may not have predicted. The DNP advanced practice nurse supports and enhances the work of the researcher, demonstrating a synergistic benefit that neither could realize in isolation.

One theoretical model that describes the process and expected outcomes of implementation and dissemination is the Donabedian model (Figure 14.1).

As Conrad and O'Dell (2014) point out by citing Fontaine and Langston, DNP programs are "forging new territory for translational science" and that "outcomes will need to be assessed in a robust manner" (p. 386). The authors submit a model to illustrate the implementation of DNP scholarly projects to improve outcomes, the *Donabedian Model of DNP Scholarly Project Outcomes* (Conrad & O'Dell, 2014, p. 388). Though specific to the context of disseminating a DNP project, the process of dissemination fits nicely into this same model (Figure 14.2).

Donabedian (1988) focuses on three main categories: structure, process, and outcomes. *Structure* refers to the quality of the attributes of an organization

FIGURE 14.1 *Donabedian Model of DNP Scholarly Project Outcomes*

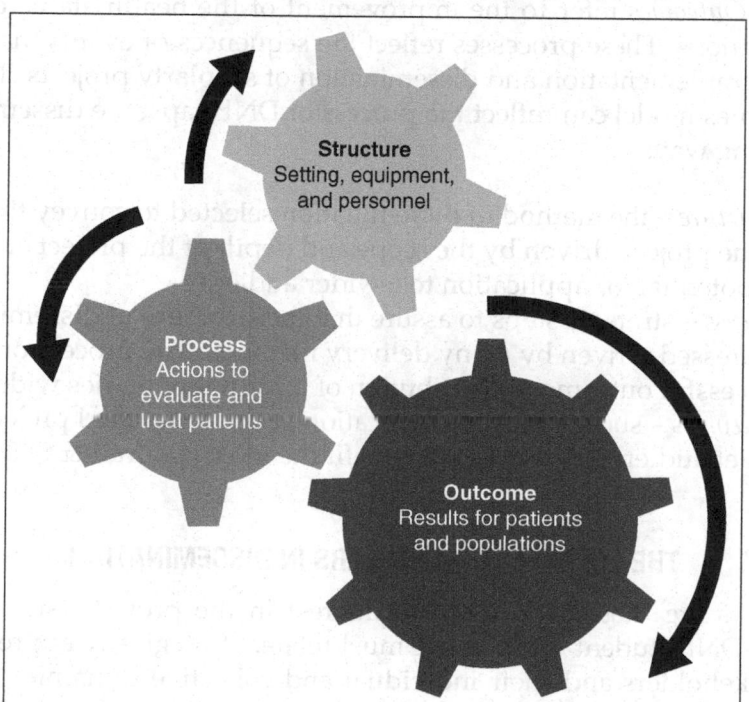

Source: Conrad & O'Dell, 2014, p. 388.

FIGURE 14.2 *Donabedian Model Application to Dissemination of Practice Scholarship*

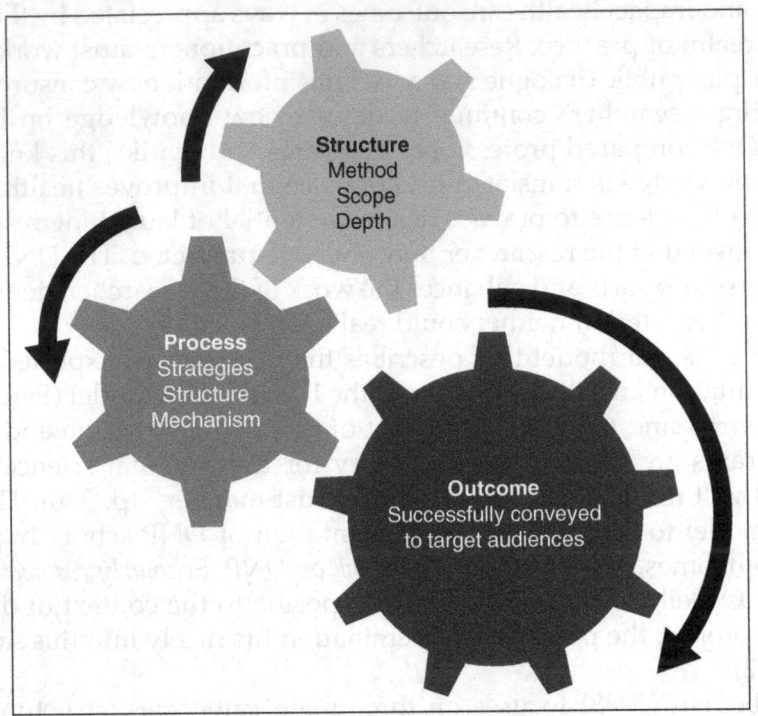

Source: Conrad & O'Dell, 2014, p. 385.

or entity. *Process* refers to how care is delivered and ultimately how quality is produced. *Outcomes* refer to the improvement of the health status of patients and populations. These processes reflect the sequences of events that lead to a successful implementation and dissemination of scholarly projects. This health care outcomes model can reflect the process of DNP capstone dissemination in the following way:

- *Structure* – the method of dissemination selected to convey the findings of the project, driven by the scope and depth of the project and its potential for application to a wider audience.
- *Process* – strategic steps to assure that the structure of dissemination is addressed, driven by many delivery methods. The process of achieving successful outcome of distribution of information varies widely.
- *Outcomes* – successful communication of the completed project to the target audience(s) that could benefit the most (Conrad & O'Dell, 2014).

THE ROLE OF STAKEHOLDERS IN DISSEMINATION

Stakeholders are those who have an interest in the project's success and to whom the DNP student or graduate must relate. Strategically appreciating the role of stakeholders and their individual and collective dynamics can help a project evolve or be destroyed. The first stakeholder, though sometimes overlooked, is the patient. The patient is the reason that a project is being developed, implemented, evaluated, and disseminated. The patient is the ultimate evaluator of the outcome. The "patient" can be defined as an individual, family (of biology or selection), aggregate population, or a specifically identified group. The patient is the ultimate customer.

Other stakeholders are incorporated at all levels of health care as well as in systems and organizations external to health care delivery systems. Not all health care is delivered or received in health care systems such as hospitals and long-term care facilities. These systems are complex and diverse, regardless of size or geographic locations. DNP scholarly practice needs to be disseminated to many levels of stakeholders, at the micro- to macrosystem level.

Medicine and nursing have declarations of professional responsibility to support and improve health care outcomes for society as a key stakeholder (American Medical Association, 2001; American Nurses Association, 2001). In tandem with this responsibility to society, the DNP advanced practice nurses are obligated to society, a key stakeholder to implement and disseminate DNP projects.

Another key stakeholder is the nursing profession. The discipline of nursing and its many professional organizations have operational standards, expectations of practice, and clinical guidelines that impact the process of DNP scholarship. These nursing organizations expect current standards to be met and are ultimately enhanced by scholarly work. The nursing profession is a critical stakeholder to consider in implementation and dissemination.

Finally, academia is a stakeholder that cannot be overlooked. The faculty and administration of DNP programs aim to have the highest level of scholarly product possible within the time frame and scope of the program. Though curricula may vary from one academic setting to another, the American Association of Colleges of Nursing (AACN) and the Center for Collegiate Nursing Education (CCNE) direct the underlying foundations for these programs (AACN, 2006). The DNP degree was created by the AACN and is evaluated by the CCNE, among other organizations, to assure quality in process and outcomes (AACN, 2006). Academia is a key stakeholder in the process of DNP project development, including implementation and dissemination.

As stakeholders and consumers of DNP project outcomes, the abovementioned stakeholders have an interest in the quality of the project. Yet none of these stakeholders have the ability to directly disseminate these outcomes. The responsibility of communicating and disseminating findings to a wider audience is the responsibility of the DNP graduate.

MECHANISMS OF DISSEMINATION

There are many ways to disseminate clinical scholarship. Categories of dissemination include professional organizations, the Internet, conferences and symposiums, continuing education offerings, collaboration with community organizations, peer-reviewed publications, consumer-driven publications, organizational policy, and legislative initiatives. These categories are not exhaustive, but do capture the majority of opportunities to disseminate findings of a DNP scholarly practice project.

Professional Organizations

The nursing profession has many organizations that reflect the diversity of the discipline. Not all professional nursing organizations lend themselves to practice scholarship. Some are dedicated to the development and dissemination of new knowledge in the form of original research. This dedication is essential to the growth of the discipline, as is the application of research to practice. Some questions to ask include:

- Does the organization represent the focus or specialty of the capstone topic?
- Is the writer a member of the organization?
- What options does the organization have to broadcast information?
    - A dedicated printed and/or online journal?
    - Annual or regional conferences?
    - A newsletter or periodical that points to the organization's web site?
- Does the organization have published standards or guidelines for practice? If so, do these guidelines lend themselves to a demonstration of a practice project?
- Does the organization provide contact information for members and nonmembers to explore the opportunity to submit a document reflecting a scholarly practice project?

Internet Dissemination

Another vehicle to disseminate scholarly practice projects is the Internet. Professional organizations maximize their efforts through websites and linkage with other organizations. When considering any web-based opportunity, one should look at how the website is connected to other organizations and entities. One web-based company dedicated to the dissemination of DNP scholarship is *Doctors of Nursing Practice, Inc.* (2014). The mission of DNP, Inc. is to improve health care outcomes by promoting and enhancing the doctoral-prepared nursing professional. The organization is dedicated to:

- Providing accurate and timely information
- Supporting, developing, and disseminating professional practice innovation
- Collaborating in a professional manner that demonstrates universal respect for others, and honesty and integrity in communications
- Responding with open discussions and dialogues that promote the evolution of advanced nursing practice and the growth of the DNP degree (DNP, Inc., 2014)

Some of the services offered by this company include a searchable listing of DNP scholarly practice projects, blogs and forums in an online community, and a bibliography and other resources that support the growth and development of the DNP-prepared nursing professional. The organization sponsors an annual conference, is supportive of regional initiatives, and collaborates with multiple professional organizations to promote the development of those persons holding a DNP degree.

There are limits to the Internet as a means of dissemination. The recipient must be actively involved in finding posted information and the Internet may not reach the intended audience. When considering an Internet-based opportunity for dissemination, the following points should be considered:

- Can the information be posted independently or must it go through a committee for approval?
- Do postings allow for interaction, feedback, and comments from viewers?
- Are blogs, list servers, and searchable databases available for viewers to explore?
- Does the web-based company broadcast to a wide audience? If so, how often?

Conferences and Symposia

Another strategy for dissemination is the submission of an abstract for presentation at a regional or national conference. Many organizations have national and regional conferences designed to enhance the caliber of practice and improve outcomes. The theme of the conference should be considered and it is ideal to be a member of the organization. One should evaluate the following in submission:

- Are guidelines and expectations for presentations clearly provided?
- Are timelines, submission expectations, and review criteria provided?
- Does the conference planning organization offer any remuneration or discounts for presenters?
- If a poster presentation, are criteria for presentation provided (dimensions if a printed poster, image size if a digital poster)?
- Is there employer support to attend the conference if the offering is selected?

Continuing Education Offerings

A benefit of continuing education offerings is sharing information to enhance the expertise of colleagues. Numerous education companies exist to address the continuing professional growth of health care professionals, often offered across health care disciplines. This transdisciplinary approach may help to disseminate the capstone results. Within the nursing profession, continuing education companies address all levels of practice. Some considerations when approaching a continuing education company may include the following questions:

- Does the company accept unsolicited submissions?
- Are expectations for submission provided in either the company's printed or online information?
- Does the diversity of the continuing education offerings provided by this company fit with the intended submission?

- Are there any expenses as a result of submitting a project for a continuing education offering?
- Is there any payment, honorarium, or royalty if the continuing education company distributes the offering?

Collaboration With Community Organizations

This option for dissemination is frequently overlooked. The content of the project must compliment and support the mission of the community organization. If there is synchronicity in efforts, the work of the DNP scholar can potentially reach a large audience while supporting the growth and development of a community organization. An initiative by an organization to improve the health or quality of life of those that it serves is an ideal collaboration for the DNP-prepared nursing professional.

Some considerations when seeking to establish contact and develop rapport with a community-based organization may include asking the following questions:

- Does the mission of the organization fit with the direction of the DNP project?
- Has the identified organization communicated a desire to collaborate with or include input from individuals and/or other organizations to further its mission?
- Does the organization have a mechanism in place to implement the results of a DNP project?
- Is the scope of the community organization local, regional, national, or international?
- What does the DNP graduate need to do to support the mission of the community-based organization?

Peer-Reviewed Publications

This mechanism for disseminating scholarly findings is perhaps the most commonly expected process in an academic setting. The caliber of a published article that is peer reviewed supports the growth and development of the discipline, a gold standard for quality. Working with colleagues to enhance writing skills can lead to successful acceptance of a manuscript (Gross & Fonteyn, 2008; Hoke & Papa, 2014; McCleary, 2008; Pearson, VanNest, & Jasinski, 2004). Some key points to consider in submitting a manuscript include:

- Select the professional publication that best reflects the direction of the scholarly project
- Review the instructions for authors to assure that the submitted manuscript meets the specifications of the journal
- Maintain communication with the journal editor to assure that all requested information has been submitted
- If changes or modifications are recommended, address each recommendation completely

Consumer-Driven Publications

Submitting to commercial publications can deliver information to the general public and to people who can directly benefit from capstone knowledge. There is a large diversity of consumer publications covering health promotion, disease-specific issues, healthy lifestyle, family living, and self-help topics. A few considerations when submitting to a publication directed at the general public include:

- Does the publication address a population that could benefit from capstone knowledge?
- What is the length of articles in selected consumer publications? Some articles are a brief two to three paragraphs, while others include articles of several pages.
- Consider reaching out to published journalists of consumer publications to review the value of a specific topic to the target population for a publication.
- Establish rapport with editorial teams, sharing expertise.

Organizational Policies, Procedures, and Protocol

When a DNP student utilizes a health care delivery system as the venue for a capstone project, existing policies, procedures, and protocols should be incorporated into the project. As a scholarly practice project is implemented, it may directly impact policies, procedures, and/or protocols of practice within an organization. If improved outcomes result from the project, the DNP graduate should advocate for change in the processes of the organization. When considering dissemination through modifying organizational processes, the following questions should be addressed:

- Do the key stakeholders involved in the implementation of the project have influence over organizational policies?
- Have the organization's existing policies, procedures, or protocols been incorporated into the project?
- Are the outcomes of the capstone of adequate value to suggest a modification or change in policy?
- Who initiates the process of policy, procedure, or protocol change?

Legislative Initiatives

The IOM (2001) charged doctoral graduates in nursing to be prepared to design, influence, and implement health care policies that frame health care financing, practice regulation, access, safety, quality, and efficacy. The AACN (2006) has identified expectations of the DNP graduate (see Table 14.1).

If these expectations are indeed realized, the interest, ability, and initiative to disseminate outcomes through the legislative and public policy arena should be a natural progression. There are many opportunities for the graduate to influence the legislative process, yet the steps needed may be slow and require

TABLE 14.1 *American Association of Colleges of Nursing: Expectations of the DNP Graduate*

Critically analyze health policy proposals, health policies, and related issues from the perspective of consumers, nursing and other health professionals, and other stakeholders in policy and public forums.

Demonstrate leadership in the development and implementation of institutional, local, state, federal, and/or international health policy.

Influence policy makers through active participation on committees, boards, or task forces at the institutional, local, state, regional, national, and/or international levels to improve health care delivery and outcomes.

Educate others, including policy makers at all levels, regarding nursing, health policy, and patient care outcomes.

Advocate for the nursing profession within the policy and health care communities.

Develop, evaluate, and provide leadership for health care policy that shapes health care financing, regulation, and delivery.

Advocate for social justice, equity, and ethical policies within all health care arenas (AACN, 2006, p. 13).

a commitment of time and effort. DNP expertise can profoundly influence legislation and policy. Approaching legislative process is one of the most influential ways to ensure dissemination of a scholarly practice project.

All of these mechanisms reflect ways to disseminate information and promote sustainability of outcomes. A project can be translated into action or can sit on the shelf, as exemplified in this case study.

CASE STUDY

Disseminate or Perish

Disseminate

Mary earned her DNP degree upon completion of a scholarly project that demonstrated the application of evidence to a change project to a microsystems change. The anticipated size of the population affected by the project was 15 to 25 patients within a particular system. The project was implemented, and over the years many more patients benefited from her efforts. She published her work and reached numerous professional colleagues who replicated or adapted her microsystem change to their respective health care delivery systems.

Perish

Joanie earned her DNP degree with a development of a document that could potentially create a change that would affect cost savings and improved outcomes for millions. The brilliance behind the document and the rigor invested in her effort won her great recognition by her colleagues and faculty. Joanie never implemented or disseminated the document. No one has been the recipient of her efforts.

CONCLUSION

A DNP project should demonstrate application of evidence to a practice question and involve measurable outcomes. These criteria reflect a DNP scholarly practice project that warrants dissemination so that others can benefit. The caliber of a DNP practice project can be evaluated by a five-point checklist, as developed by Waldrup (2013). The five points include:

E = Enhances health outcomes (patient, system, or policy)
C = Culmination of practice inquiry
P = Partnerships
I = Implementation (translating/applying evidence into practice)
E = Evaluate (Waldrup, 2013)

If these five criteria are met, a DNP scholarly project outcome is present. Having completed the scholastic rigor of demonstrating an evidence-based health care outcome, the final step must be the dissemination.

REFERENCES

American Association of Colleges of Nursing. (2006). *The essentials of doctoral education for advanced nursing practice.* Washington, DC: Author. Retrieved from http://www .aacn.nche.edu/publications/position/dnpessentials.pdf

American Medical Association. (2001). *Declaration of professional responsibility: Medicine's social contract with humanity.* Retrieved from http://www.ama-assn.org/ resources/doc/ethics/decofprofessional.pdf

American Nurses Association. (2001). *Code of ethics for nurses.* Retrieved from http:// www.nursingworld.org/codeofethics

Conrad, D., & O'Dell, D. (2014). The rest of the story—evaluating the doctor of nursing practice. In K. J. Moran, R. Burson, & D. Conrad (Eds.), *The doctor of nursing practice scholarly project: A framework for success* (pp. 385–410). Burlington, MA: Jones & Bartlett.

Doctors of Nursing Practice, Inc. (2014). *About us.* Retrieved from http://www.doctor-sofnursingpractice.org/aboutus.html

Donabedian, A. (1988). Quality assessment and assurance: Unity of purpose, diversity of means. *Inquiry, 25*(1), 173–192.

Eagleman, D. M. (2013). Why public dissemination of science matters: A manifesto. *The Journal of Neuroscience, 33*(30), 12147–12149. doi:10.1523/JNEUROSCI. 2556-13.2013

Gross, A. M., & Fonteyn, M. E. (2008). Turn your presentation into a published manuscript. *American Journal of Nursing, 108*(10), 85–87. doi:10.1097/01.NAJ.0000337 747.37719.86

Hoke, L. M., & Papa, A. M. (2014). Increasing the odds, using peer review promotes successful abstract submission. *Clinical Nurse Specialist, 28*(1), 46–55. doi:10.1097/ NUR.0000000000000019

Health Services Research Information Center. (2014). *Dissemination and implementation science.* National Information Center on Health Services Research and Health Care

Technology. Retrieved from http://www.nlm.nih.gov/hsrinfo/implementation_science.html

Institutes of Medicine. (2001). *Crossing the quality chasm: A new health system for the 21st century.* Washington, DC: The National Academies Press. Retrieved from http://www.nap.edu/catalog.php?record_id=10027

McCleary, L. (2008). Drawing support from a writing group. *Nursing, 38*(9), 46–47. doi:10.1097/01.NURSE.0000334648.74831.ee

Pearson, J. A., VanNest, R. L., & Jasinski, D. M. (2004). Promoting publication by producing a student journal. *Nurse Educator, 29*(2), 68–70.

U.S. Department of Health and Human Services, National Institutes of Health, Office of Behavioral and Social Sciences Research. (2013). *Dissemination and implementation.* Retrieved from http://obssr.od.nih.gov/scientific_areas/translation/dissemination_and_implementation/index.aspx

Waldrup, J. (2013, November 8). *EC as PIE: Five check points for determining quality in DNP final projects.* Presented at the Drexel Advanced Practice and Doctoral Education Conference, Baltimore, MD.

Index

AARP, 104
academia, 175
Academic Chronic Care Collaborative
    (ACCC), 55, 57
    University of Kentucky, 59, 62, 63
accreditation
    CCNE, 19
    LACE, 11
Accreditation Commission for Education
    in Nursing (ACEN), 91
Advanced Emergency Nursing Journal, The, 75
Advanced practice nursing, 33, 100, 131, 133
advanced practice psychiatric nurses
    (APPNs), 34, 36, 41
advanced practice registered nurses
    (APRNs), 4, 5, 11, 12, 17, 18, 19, 23,
    34, 100, 101
Agency for Healthcare Research and
    Quality (AHRQ), 84
allocative efficiency, 101
American Academy of Nurse Practitioners
    (AANP), 104
American Association of Birth Centers
    (AABC), 80, 82, 84
American Association of Colleges of
    Nursing (AACN), 10, 31, 45, 67,
    79, 87, 89, 91, 99, 103, 107, 117,
    131, 175
    DNP graduate, expectations of, 180
    *Essentials of Doctoral Education for
    Advanced Nursing Practice, The*, 4, 5–6,
    18, 33, 132, 139–145, 163, 165
    Nursing Outlook, 6
    *Position Statement on the Practice Doctorate
    in Nursing*, 4, 18
American Board of Comprehensive Care
    (ABCC), 157
    certification exam, 12

American College of Nurse–Midwives
    (ACNM), 47, 48, 51
    Life-Saving Skills series, 112
American Organization of Nurse Executives
    (AONE), 76
American Public Health Association
    (APHA), 104
Anderson, Barbara A., 45, 67, 79, 99, 107, 131
appendix, in case narrative
    writing, 156–157
Association of American Medical Colleges
    (AAMC), 57

bachelor's of science in nursing to doctor
    of nursing (BSN-DNP), 6, 17–29
    national movement toward, 18–19
    program development, 19–29
        clinical sites and project
        development, 23–25
        clinical translation of research, 20–21
        program length, 21–23
        translational research, 25–29
Beck Youth Depression Inventory, 40
birth center care, consumer demand for, 80
birth center costs, 81
Blue Cross Blue Shield of Michigan
    Foundation Collaboration, 84
Brief Cognitive-Behavioral COPE Intervention
    for Depressed Adolescents: Outcomes
    and Feasibility of Delivery in 30-Minute
    Outpatient Visits, The, 34
burning clinical question in PICOT
    format, 36–37
burnout (BO), 68, 71
    as barrier to nurse–midwives, 45–51
        capstone focus, 45
        capstone project, 47–51
        literature review, 46–47

Printed in the United States
By Bookmasters